Why Are You Working Harder And Making Less Money?

11 Habits

of Highly Successful Dentists

Dr. John Meis

Publisher: The Team Training Institute, www.TheTeamTrainingInstitute.com

ISBN: 1719228280

ISBN-13: 9781719228282

Free Resources Just For Book Readers!

Because this topic is so important to the Dental Community and because everyone learns differently, we have created a special area for readers of this book.

The great news is access to this area is completely free.

You can register and receive free access at…

www.11HabitsToolkit.com

Here's what you will find when you register for your free access…

* All of the downloadable resources mentioned throughout the book.

* 3 advanced video trainings on the 11 Secrets of Highly Successful Dentists

* BONUS Video Training: Why What Got You To Where You Are Today Won't Get You To Where You Want To Go Tomorrow

Simply register to receive free access at:

www.11HabitsToolkit.com

Why Are You Working Harder and Making Less Money?

Dedication

This book is dedicated to the many people whose wisdom and ideas inspired the words on the following pages.

Firstly, my family. My wife Kelly who covered our home fort while I was on countless calls and traveling to many amazing practices (270 at current count). Her loving support is in every word. My daughters, Samantha and Stacy, who are amazing women entrepreneurs that challenge and inspire me more each day. Samantha would be happy to offer you an amazing curated coffee experience at mistobox.com. Stacy is marketing strategist at stacyrust.com who can help you grow your business.

Secondly, my "right hand," Heather Driscoll. She has been along for this learning journey since Day 1. Her intelligence, knowledge, passion, kindness, and work ethic are second to none. I am the luckiest man alive to have her as a friend, confidant, co-worker, and partner. Thanks also to the love of her life, husband Aric Wiese, whose support has been instrumental.

Thirdly, my brain-trust the "Elite Mastermind." These mentors patiently taught me how to be a better clinician and practice owner. I am forever grateful to these amazing dentists: Roger Abbott, David Ahearn, Mike Ariana, Kelly Bridenstine, Gary Cameron, John Evanish, Mitchel Friedman, David Gage, Brian Gilbert, Steve Johnson, George Loftus, Vince Monticciolo, Wayne Mortenson, Dave Neumeister, Tom Peltzer, Roy Smith, Bret Tobler, Chuck Tozzer, and Paul Weyman.

And lastly, Darcy Juarez without whose talent and persistence this book would still be a set of ideas in my head.

TABLE OF CONTENTS

TABLE OF CONTENTS

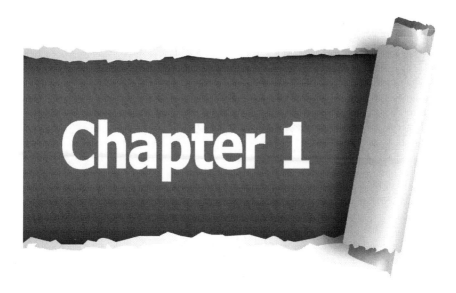

Why Are You Working Harder and Making Less Money?

Dentistry has changed. It used to be that you could open up a practice and patients would come to you because you were a good dentist. Patients paid their bills, and as a dentist, we made a pretty good living. We could send our kids to good schools, drive a nice car, play golf on Wednesday afternoons, and even have a summer home to relax at on weekends.

Boy have times changed … it's no longer enough to just be a good dentist. It's no longer enough to just open up a practice. It's no longer feasible (for most) to be a fee-for-service practice. Which means we have to learn how to play the insurance game, we have to be open in the evenings,

1

and weekend. We now have to treat our practice like a business and that was the biggest breakthrough I discovered.

When I started treating my practice like a business and I focused on solving business problems (not just dental problems) my practice took off. I was able to serve more patients and provide better care while creating a better life for my family, my team and their families.

My goal, in writing this book is to show you the secrets that I have learned over 30+ years in dentistry that allowed me to go from earning an income to creating wealth. From working to directing. From worry and competition to peace of mind. If you follow this blueprint, you can go from where you are today to something new and completely transformational … a way to live a bigger life now and a brighter future tomorrow.

If you feel like you are already behind schedule to retire (or want to ensure that you never fall behind), if you have a paycheck but want profits, if you have an income but want wealth, if you have a job but want a business, or if you have a lifestyle but want security, then this is vital information for you.

The secret lies with just 3 keys…

Key #1: Utilize the 11 habits of highly successful dentists.

Key #2: Create a culture of high productivity, providing patients with what they want, and providing a world-class patient experience.

Key #3: Understand that the only practice worth owning is a practice worth selling.

The 11 habits of highly successful dentists. These habits can all be learned, so if you are motivated to achieve more from your practice and want a self-managing dental practice that will give you more time, money and freedom, then you are in the right place.

Creating a culture of high productivity, providing patients with what they want while providing a world-class patient experience will provide you with the revenue and income to create the practice of your dreams. It's not unusual for clients to tell me that they have doubled their production in just 12 short months.

With that, they are able to take 2 weeks to go on mission trips to Africa to provide dental care to those who have never seen a toothbrush. They are single-handily providing supplies and time to human-trafficking survivors by opening up shelters. I outline the processes to double your production my book *The Ultimate Guide to Doubling Your*

Dental Practice Production...How to Build an Unstoppable Dental Practice With the Freedom to Enjoy It!

And lastly, those who have created the practice of their dreams understand that the only practice worth owning is a practice worth selling. Dentists who create a practice worth selling having ambitions big enough to pull them beyond their current capabilities and into bigger, brighter futures.

There is an end for all of us, and when you practice with that end in mind – you build a practice that will provide for your family long after you decide to retire.

How do I know all of this? Because unlike anyone else giving you advice on how to achieve financial freedom as a dentist, I have actually done it. I did it by learning these 11 habits, then building an amazing practice, and then by learning how to buy, build, and sell practices.

As a partner and leader of development, and later as President, I guided a groups practice growth from 50 to 120 locations. Then I sold my interest for more than 10 times what I could have hoped to earn as a dentist. Now, you don't have to aspire to run 120 offices, as I did. It's the principles that matter regardless of how big you want your enterprise to grow.

I have done a lot right but I have done a lot more wrong. After nearly 30 years I discovered how to grow your practice with zero special advantages. And it all started when I learned, what I have coined as 'The 11 habits of highly successful dentists.'

How I Discovered The 11 Habits of Highly Successful Dentists

Let me tell you a little bit about how I came to discover these 11 habits. And it begins with my start in dentistry. I started in 1986, practicing in a small town in Iowa in the depths of the farm crisis of the mid-'80s.

If you remember, at that time, all the family farms were failing; there was no credit to be had; even the banks were failing. It was awful. The price of corn was 99 cents a bushel. It hadn't been that low since the Great Depression. It was a very tough time to get started, and I had a very lean start.

But I had an opportunity to build up a little practice, but it was going to have to be in the midst of this very difficult time. And by little practice, I mean little.

Now, when I look back at it, I have to admit it was a little dump – but it was mine – and I was very proud of it because it represented all my hopes and dreams and it was mine to build (or as I came to learn) mine to destroy.

Then one night I woke up at 2:37 a.m. I remember it like it was yesterday, with pain, like I had never felt before. I quickly knew that something was wrong – very wrong. I had a practice I had just purchased with the intent of building. My health started to deteriorate. The chest pain led to fatigue, which led to more pain and fatigue. I seemed to be getting sicker and sicker.

It took what seemed like an eternity for the doctors to diagnose me with cardiomyopathy (which is an autoimmune disease of the heart). I sat in the doctor's office after they told me, and all I could think about was my family … I had added to my debt by buying a practice; I had my family depending on me, my staff depending on me, my patients depending on me. What was going to happen to all of them?

I was one of the lucky ones. Cardiomyopathy leads to heart failure, and heart failure leads to a transplant or death. Luckily for me, immune suppressants were effective, and over the course of the year, the pain stopped and the fatigue resolved. I have been symptom-free for almost 30 years. But the terrified feeling that I had sitting in that doctor's office 30 years ago has never left me; instead, it had a profound effect on me in several ways. I became obsessed with financial security for my family. I didn't need much, but I wanted my family to be safe and secure, should it ever come back.

I started taking all kinds of clinical courses – everything that everyone recommended (and remember this was in the 1990s); all of the courses at The Dawson Academy, all the courses at Frank Spear's group. I took Ross Nash's continuum. I went to the MISCH Institute, got my FAGD, etc.

I learned how to do clinical dentistry well. I learned from some of the very best people, and I'm glad I did because it made me a better dentist and allowed me to treat more cases and more complex cases. But at the end of 4-5 years of taking courses, I was still very, very frustrated because I wasn't any closer to financial security than I had been when I started. And finding financial security was the whole reason I wanted to learn from the very best dentists.

I was now growing frustrated and ever more anxious about finances

I started looking for consultants to help me with the business side of the practice. One of these consultants invited me to a conference in Phoenix; it was a group of their bigger clients who were sharing all the things that were working in their practices.

I had been in groups with dentists before, and I immediately knew that something was different with this group. They were looking at their dental practices differently than I was. They were interested in doing fantastic dentistry and serving their patients and serving their teams, **but** they're also interested in running their practice as a **business**. They were way ahead of where I was in finding financial freedom.

I was beginning to understand it. If you want to learn how to play basketball, you don't ask a football player; you ask a basketball player. If you want to learn how to help your practices' business improve, you talk to the people that have a really good, well-run business side of their practices.

I had spent all this time on clinical education to learn to become more financially secure, but I was learning from the wrong people. (note: *Be careful about who you learn things from.*)

Once this light bulb went off, I put together a group of dentists that all had successful practices, most were way bigger than mine. They were extremely financially successful – I still refer to them as My Brain Trust. At the time, it was called the Apogee's Elite Mastermind Group.

I learned a tremendous amount from these very brilliant guys. This learning became the basis for the 11 habits disclosed in this book. We all hear lots of brilliant ideas from tons of brilliant people. What made the difference for me was that I went to work and rapidly applied these learnings to my practice. (What I did to triple my practice in just four short years is detailed in my training "How to Double Your Production Starting Tomorrow" which is available through www.TheTeamTrainingInstitute.com)

My Practice Tripled in
4 Short Years

It was no small feat to triple in four years; I had grown a relatively big practice by this point. And knowing what I know now, I could have cut that time down to just two years. But I wasn't done there; I then merged that practice with another group, and that practice has now grown to 12 locations.

But it all started when I studied these **successful** dentists. I intentionally picked these people *because* of their success.

But how do you define success?

Success is not the same for one person as it is for another. It was a very diverse group. One of the guys in there had an office with two operatories. All he did was high fee large case dentistry. Small practice numbers but he only did the type of dentistry that he enjoyed. He achieved his definition of success.

Another member was in the denture model. Within his general practice, he was making a lot of dentures in a highly efficient manner. There were several members whose strategy included sedation. Most of the members were very, very productive. The interesting thing about this group of extremely talented and financially successful people is that they didn't realize that they were doing anything unique or special.

They were all at the top of our profession.

Most of them were financially far more successful than I was.

After digesting what I learned from these guys…I realized that they were not only **doing** things differently, they were **thinking** differently. I started to study what was different and refine those things into the traits, habits, and thoughts that every single one of them possessed.

The 11 Habits of Highly Successful Dentists

These 11 habits and thought processes are what separated the practices which were good in quality care and businesses from those who were just good dentists like those I had met in so many of all the clinical courses I had taken.

The 11 habits/mind-sets were:

1. Create a Vision and Goals

2. Become Team Oriented
3. Instill Discipline
4. Become Service Oriented
5. Know Your Statistics
6. Be Aware of Capacity
7. Always Be (Smartly) Marketing
8. Know the Technology Rules
9. Wants, Needs, Wants
10. Understand Research and Development
11. Winning the Mental Game

I relayed it all back to the group, and they were astounded. They then encouraged me to teach this to others. They opened my eyes to the fact that what I had synthesized from studying all of them were keys to business success in dentistry that no one else was teaching.

I started by teaching these 11 habits, which are mind-sets or behaviors that I found in every successful dentist who had built a very financially and secure practice.

These principles are different than any I had come upon in dental school.

Before we dive in, I want you to know something; these are not my original ideas. In fact, I've only had three original ideas in my life, and two of them were really bad ideas… ha-ha. I was very fortunate that I had these wonderful people who helped me learn. *(This is another lesson in and of itself – there are very few original ideas, but there are so many great ideas that you can take from both inside and outside of dentistry that will skyrocket your practice.)*

I have become very successful through a simple process. I learn from other people. I learn from other people's uniqueness. I understand what makes them successful. I break that down into the simplest steps, and I find an easy way for people to understand those simple steps. With insight to over 180 practices, if I simply pay attention, I get 180 years of experience every single year. I have a great opportunity to learn a great deal and to share that knowledge.

So let's get started ...

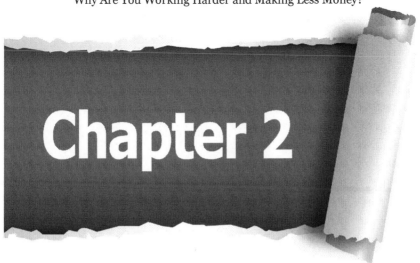

Chapter 2

Why a Vision With Goals Can Foreshadow Your Revenue

Habit #1: Create Vision and Goals

When I interview a doctor about their practice, I ask them about where their practice is going. Based on the answer I get, I can come pretty close to determining how well the practice is doing. Practices that are doing extremely well have a very clear and concise answer to where their practice is going.

Most dentists haven't seriously considered or thought about vision and goals, not for themselves, and not for their teams. Less than 4% have written goals that they review weekly.

Highly successful dentists have a very, very different way of looking at vision and goals. The most successful dentists can articulate their vision and can recite their main goals without notes.

For some, their vision may have something to do with their business model. For instance, one elite mastermind member's office had two operatories; his vision was to do comprehensive restored dentistry on every patient. That's it. He can say it very succinctly, and you know immediately what he was saying. He has very, very clear vision.

When you have a clear vision, you know what to spend your time developing, you know what to spend your time learning, and you know what's more import than anything else. You also know what <u>not</u> to spend time doing. The clarity of vision is critically important.

Realistically, pretty much every dentist that I talk to can give me *some* idea of what their vision is. I'm involved in a lot of dental mergers and acquisitions. I get the opportunity to talk to people who are purchasing practices, and I often ask them to describe their vision.

The response goes something like this, "*Uh....*" (long pause followed by stumbling over words.) They are trying to formulate an answer. That's not having a clearly defined vision and having it set up in a way that you can describe it quickly and simply.

The leader of the largest practice in the Elite Mastermind understood how important it is to have clarity about the vision. When asked, he could very clearly explain it.

"A legacy model of building practice, after practice, after practice. Having dentists invest in the growth and having a model of a group practice that provides the advantage of a large group, yet had the feel of a smaller practice. Utilizing dentist ownership so that the practice will endure."

In this model, the faces would change, but the company would endure from one generation to the next.

A clearly defined vision is very, very important. The ability to articulate it well is even more so. Can you describe your vision in a way that people understand who you are and what you do?

The "Jay Leno" Test

Does your team understand what your vision is? When I go into a practice, trying to assess the quality and the strength of the team and the strength of the leader, I use what I call the Jay Leno test.

The Jay Leno test is this. Those of you who watched the Jay Leno show remember that he used to go out on the street often to a shopping area in Los Angeles where he would ask people random questions.

Questions like, "Who is the vice president of the United States?" They were usually ridiculously easy questions, and it was amazing and quite funny that so many people had no idea what the answer was to such easy questions.

I've used the Jay Leno test when I'm testing a team and the leadership of that team. I'll go in and ask the question, "Where do you see this practice being in five years? Where is this practice headed?"

On a well led team, they'll be able to tell you exactly where it's going because they know the vision and they know how to describe it to people.

I can tell you hearing a dental team who can provide a clear answer to this vision question is very rare. Most of the time, when asked that question, the person will look at you as if they're looking into the surface of the sun.

They'll have this blank stare because they won't have any idea how to answer that question. No one has ever explained it to them or helped them learn how to say it to other people. The ability to communicate your vision is easy to do and worth the effort.

The Uninformed Test

The next is the uninformed test. The uninformed test is simply this:

If you didn't know anything about the practice, didn't know anything about the people and you heard the vision, would you understand what it meant?

The easiest way to do this is to hop on to somebody's website. Can you tell what their vision is? Can you tell where that practice is heading? Can you tell what to expect when you get there? If you can't, it does not pass the uninformed test.

To pass the uninformed test: have a clear vision, be able to articulate it yourself, have your team be able to understand it and articulate it themselves, and have it worded in a way that the general public will understand who you are and where you're going.

Having a clear vision and the ability to articulate it well is one of the keys to practice success.

Goals

When I work with practices, the first question I ask is, "Can I see your goals?"

How many practices do you think have written goals?

It is shocking to me how very, very, very few practices have written goals. If you don't have written goals, all you have is a bunch of dreams.

Key to Goal Setting

It is imperative that you have a very clear vision in below communicate it clearly before setting your goals. Your vision must:

- Resonate with patients
- Resonate with your team
- Be authentic to you

I highly recommend that you have a very disciplined planning process to set goals. Most often I observed practices that have a very weak planning process. These are some of the most common problems that I see:

- The practice goals are vague
- Practice goals don't have specific dates for completion
- The goals are unattainable due to a goal itself or the time allotted to complete it
- There are no measurable outcomes specified
- Goals are relevant to the vision

The planning process I teach is very simple yet extremely effective. It engages the team. It challenges the leaders. It creates clarity, connection, and confidence.

The planning process begins with the team being given a questionnaire. The questionnaire is to be filled out off-site and in private and should be brought to the next team meeting. The questionnaire asks these six questions:

- What should we do to improve the patient experience?
- What should we do to increase our treatment capabilities?
- What should we do to develop our team?
- What should we do to upgrade or upkeep our facility?
- What should we do to improve our marketing, promotion, and patient attraction?
- What should we do to increase revenue and decrease costs?

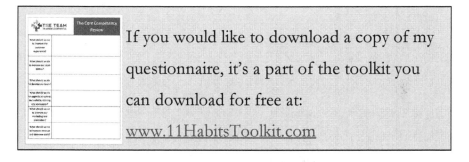

If you would like to download a copy of my questionnaire, it's a part of the toolkit you can download for free at:

www.11HabitsToolkit.com

The next full team meeting should be spent discussing what people have written on their sheets. I would take each question and ask the team to share their answers. Write the answers on a white board or flipchart. Lead the team to prioritize which of the items would be most impactful if they were implemented.

Armed with a good understanding of what is most important to the team, you are prepared to begin the next step of the planning process. The process begins with the leadership team; however, you define that, setting very general 5 year goals and ends with a highly specific plan for the next quarter. This plan, called the 90 Day Sprint, identifies 7-12 strategic projects and specifies who is responsible for what.

We begin with a five-year projection of revenues. For each of the next five years determine what level of revenue would make you feel happy with your progress. After watching dozens of teams follow the process, I know the most teams over estimate what they can accomplish in the short term and underestimate what is possible in the long term. If the five-year number doesn't scare you more than a little bit … it is too low.

Next, look specifically at the three-year revenue. As a team, imagine what would need to be in place to hit that number. Perhaps you'll need more. Which often means you'll need better recruiting and training systems. Maybe you'll need additional providers. Maybe you'll need multiple locations. Think through what will have to change and improve to hit that three-year number. Once the picture is clear on what your practice will look like in three years it is time to move to the next step.

Repeat the process for one-year revenue. Answer the question what will have to be true by the end of this year to be on track to hit that three-year image. You now have a clear vision of what things look like a year from now.

The rubber meets the road at the next step. Answer the question, "what do we have to do in the next 90 days to achieve that one year vision?" Using the entire team's input, the leadership team's input, and your own good judgment, identify specifically the 7-12 projects that need to be done in the next 90 days in order to reach the one year vision.

At this point you have the "what" figured out, the "when" is pre-determined (90 days), the "who" is still a question mark. Assign, as a group, <u>one</u> person to be responsible for completing each of the 7-12 projects. Many people may be involved with each project but only one person is responsible.

But I don't stop with the business planning….

The Personal Planning Process

I have a **personal planning process** that's very similar.

One difference, I find I get more creative if I get out of my usual environment. I get away. I don't even do it in my home city.

I will get out of town. I'll hole up in a place that's private and quiet with few distractions.

I will spend the whole day, and I will first of all celebrate the things that I got done. Once I celebrate the accomplishments, I spend time being grateful for what I accomplished. Grateful especially for the people that helped me make it happen.

I next review where I'm going to be three years from now. Even though I did it 90 days before, I still go back to the same discipline every time.

Most of us set goals and make plans but never get everything done; we don't accomplish everything we set out to achieve.

Now, my three-year goals don't change every time, so from one 90-day period to another 90-day period, they may not have changed, but I am still rethinking it. I'm still getting it into my brain.

Amazing things happen when you put a three-year goal out there that's larger than you can grasp … larger than you think you can accomplish.

What happens is your brain goes to work on it. If you're committed to it, you've written it down, you've got a date, your brain automatically starts working on it. It can't help not to.

Your goal is "I'm going to get my practice to $2 million next year." If you are truly committed to whatever it takes to get there, your brain will go to work.

Your Brain Works on It

Now your brain starts to work on it.

- It works on it when you're sleeping.
- It works on it when you're driving.
- It works on it when you're in the shower.
- It works on it when you're doing stuff you enjoy.
- It works on it when you're exercising.
- It works on it all the time in the background.

It's chugging away, figuring out how to do it.

Making Improvements

I go through the three-year goals, I go through my one-year goals, and I go through what I need to accomplish in the next 90 days and fill out my 90-day sprint sheet that I keep on me at all times.

I will pick out areas of my life that I want to improve on, so I always start with my family ... "What can I do to improve the relationships with my family and friends?" I always start there.

Then I start thinking about the different areas of the businesses that I'm involved in. I do it every quarter. I never fail to do this process, and the process never fails me.

Every Monday, I look at the plan and my 90-day sprint. I refresh my memory. I pull it out. I have a big sheet that it's all written on. I look at it. It refreshes my memory.

It refreshes my excitement about the goals, and then I go to work.

As you begin the planning process, you will find that it's awkward at first because it's not something that we typically do. Don't be alarmed. This isn't the only effective method. "How" you do it isn't as important as "that" you do it.

Your three-year goal should be bigger than you will imagine accomplishing.

When you combine your business goal setting with your personal planning process, you can see amazing things start to happen!

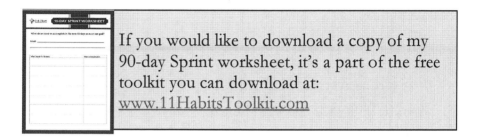

If you would like to download a copy of my 90-day Sprint worksheet, it's a part of the free toolkit you can download at:
www.11HabitsToolkit.com

I'm going to talk about specific practices from my "Brain Trust." I'm going to disguise them a little bit so that I don't embarrass these guys too much.

Goal: Maximizing **Income**

I'm going to talk about Dr. #1. first. His main goal was to **maximize his income.**

Dr. #1 wanted a practice that served a lot of patients. He wanted to do a lot of treatment with a lot of patients going through the practice. He was serving all ends of demographic spectrum with good dentistry.

His practice reached the highest personal production of a single doctor in a single month of which I'm aware. This doctor did $345,0000 in production in one month. That's just him. That's not the whole practice. That's not hygiene, that's not associates. There were associates, and there was hygiene in the practice, but that $345,000 was just him. That's a record that is absolutely hard for me to imagine hitting, but he did.

He was very, very clear on what the vision was, he was very clear on what his goals were, and his goals had very specific numbers. They had goals for every part of the practice. Their break room had whiteboards covering every wall. All the whiteboards had goals written on them. The numbers, the progress towards those goals, and very clearly stated who is responsible for the goal.

When it comes to a goal, you can have many people working on the goal, but you can only have one person responsible. (It's a very, very important concept learned the hard way myself.) One of the smart guys that I worked with had an expression that I loved, "The fastest way to starve a horse is to put two people in charge of feeding it."

People start to laugh when I say that because they can picture what will happen. One person thinks the other person is doing it and the other one thinks the other one's doing it, and the horse goes hungry.

This office created a set of tactics to carry out their goals and to reach their vision. For instance;

- Sedation Dentistry. Sedation dentistry allows you to do a large amount of dentistry in a single appointment, allows you to treat people that are highly fearful, a lot of surgical care as well as other kinds of care.

- "Cherry-Picking" which means the high-producing doctor did all the crown and bridge. He had associate doctors that did the simpler procedures, and he did the more complex. He did the surgeries. Cherry-picking allowed him to maximize his production.

Let's look closer at both Sedation and Cherry Picking:

Sedation Dentistry

If you are not doing sedation in your offices right now, sedation has some effects on the practice that you may not fully appreciate.

What happens with sedation is you begin to attract a different type of patient. Sedation patients often, not always, are high-fear patients.

They often have avoided dentistry for a long time. Maybe five years. Maybe ten. Maybe more.

If someone avoids dentistry for ten years, the condition of their mouth is going to be bad.

Now, we all have really bad mouths walking into our practices all the time. We see train wrecks all the time.

The person with anxiety about dentistry that has a trainwreck mouth has something different, and it's very unique.

People who have anxiety are usually not anxious about just one thing. They're usually anxious about a lot of things.

Some of the things that anxiety patients are scared about include:

- Needles.
- The drill – the feeling, the vibration.
- Pain.
- Gagging.
- The enclosed room – being claustrophobic.
- People hovering over them.

Many also have a fear of how much it's going to cost.

The way I like to describe or think about anxiety is like the brakes in the brain turn off; so, you have a thought, it raises your anxiety level. If you don't have anxiety about it, your brain applies the brakes and it stops.

If you do have anxiety, you think about the thought. It makes you more anxious. You think about it some more; you get more anxious, more anxious, and more anxious.

Many people can think of situations where they have something that they're focusing on and focusing on, and it's raising and raising their anxiety level.

Why the sedation train wreck patient is different is that they have already been anxious about how much it's going to cost. They've already built that expected cost up and up and up and up and up.

Then, when you tell them how much it's going to cost, it's amazing to me how frequently they say, "Is that all? I thought it was going to be worse."

I don't know about you, but none of my other patients ever said that. None. That's why sedation has a profound impact.

- First of all, your case acceptance is higher.

- Secondly, the case size is bigger.

Then there's productivity per hour. If you are doing sedation, you're not doing a few procedures and then having them come back and doing a few more procedures. You're doing a whole bunch at one time.

And that is clinically efficient. There is no waste of time. There's no room turnover.

It's cost-efficient and time-efficient. That's why sedation has been such a successful strategy.

Now, if you're not doing sedation, one of the things I will tell you is that you won't find a lot of sedation patients in your practice now.

The sedation patients aren't in anybody's practice. They're not in yours, and they're not in anybody else's either.

These are people floating around that are searching for a solution to a very, very serious problem and haven't taken any action.

A couple of other things about sedation patients. Many of them have unique personalities.

As I said, we all have some anxiety about some things; but you're going to meet some real characters when you do sedation. In fact, they can be challenging to work with at first.

But the truth is, when you help them, they are the most grateful patients that you can have.

When you finish their treatment, they cry. They hug you. They smile and tell you, "I haven't been able to smile in seven years. I've been embarrassed about my teeth, and my life is going to be different now."

Can you imagine not being able to smile? What must that do to our brains if we couldn't smile? That is so awful. I can't even imagine it.

Sedation patients are so grateful, I found it to be very personally rewarding to help them. It was hard work, though. Sedation does not make the treatment easier for the dentist. In fact, it's more difficult. But it does make it a lot easier for the patient.

Cherry-Picking

**Cherry-picking is not a strategy for everybody. Unless you want a good deal of dentist turnover, you need to have it be a good deal for the associate dentists. In this case, the dentist and his associate dentists were all very busy. They all made a very good living because they provided a great deal of service to patients.

He built a team of people all around him so that he could reach his goal of treating a lot of people and having very high personal production. The team included assistants, hygienists, associate dentists, anesthesiologists, and endodontists.

He was an extremely effective delegator (more about delegation later.)

The results? He was the most productive dentist that I've heard of, and he built this practice into an absolutely mammoth practice, sold the practice for a high seven-figure price tag, and went into retirement where he was a complete and utter failure – not because he ran out of money, but because he wasn't ready to live the 'retirement' lifestyle. There was still so much that he wanted to do in life… and that's a great place to be in your life. Where you get to choose if you want to work or not work, where you get to do something just because you love to do it.

Now, is cherry-picking a strategy that I recommend? It's fraught with some peril because, for the dentist that is doing all of the less productive work, it may not be very professionally satisfying for them.

As far as sustainability, that's a challenge because the dentist who's getting cherry-picked may decide that that's not very fulfilling and may not stick around very long. If you're in an area where it's hard to recruit dentists, this strategy may not be the wisest.

If you're in some places where dentists are plentiful, this is a strategy that might be okay for you. You must be able to survive with a lot of associate turnover.

Delegation

What Dr. #1 did very well, was he decided that he was going to do dentistry. He was going to do as much dentistry as he possibly could, and all the other stuff in the practice he wasn't going to do.

Everything else was delegated. He had a clinical manager who managed the practice. They would meet every day for five minutes so he could give her direction. Other than that, all this mental energy was on the practice of dentistry.

Now, what I see in practices that don't reach this level is the dentist is doing everything … they are into the supplies, into the marketing, hiring, firing, training, and all the other ancillary things that the dentist doesn't have to do.

Dr. #1 eliminated all of that. He doesn't do any of it. None.

He saves every bit of his time, every bit of his mental energy to be treating patients because that's where he can be the most effective and the most productive.

He has developed an amazing team that does all of it.

He worked 16 days and he would take one long weekend a month. To help maintain his mental energy on those weekends, he would travel internationally. He's been all over the world to see all kinds of interesting places; travel rejuvenates him.

While I didn't cherry-pick when I practiced, I did use most of Dr. #1's other tactics.

Imagine if you became a better delegator, how much more productive you could be.

Are you burning time and mental energy on things that aren't producing dentistry?

The big lesson that I learned from Dr. #1 was to focus my time and energy. Let's look at some more examples of specific goals on another style of practice...

Goal: High End, Low Volume

We're going to move to Dr. #2. His goal was completely different. His goal was to have a high-end, low-volume practice.

His office was very simple; it had three ops, but they only needed two.

Every single patient received a comprehensive examination and recommendations. Most needed extensive restorative dentistry. His goal was what he called complete and ideal dentistry.

If patients weren't going to accept ideal dentistry, they didn't belong in his practice.

Over time - and it took a long time, he built a referral-only practice that was doing this low-volume, high-end dentistry. For him, it was perfect. It was exactly what he dreamed of, exactly what he wanted, and he was able to build this practice to the point that he was able to retire in his mid-60s.

Did he have huge nest egg? No, didn't have it, didn't need it, didn't want it. He was completely happy and completely successful with his model.

He had a very clear vision, he had very clear goals, and he had very clear tactics on how to get there.

***Note: these kinds of practices were absolutely crushed in the economic downturn because there was not a flow of regular patients. Most of his patients are doing mainly elective care. Patients willingness to do elective care varies with their confidence in their financial well-being. I warn you, this is a tough model to make work. It's very fragile. It's extremely risky, it was what Dr. #2 wanted, and he made it happen. He did a great job.

Goal: Maximize Wealth Creation

Next doctor is Dr. #3. His goal was to maximize wealth creation for himself and other doctors. He was looking at not only the income side of it, but also building the worth of the enterprise.

He had great clarity of vision compared to most other dentists I've worked with. He could tell you exactly what his practice model was and exactly where they were going to be.

When this practice was at $5 million in collections per year, he said, "*In three years, I want to be at $15 million.*"

That seems very hard to grasp... almost unbelievable. How do you double something that big in three years?

Well, they did it in just a little over 2 ½ years.

The practice has now many locations. Today, he has the largest net worth of any of the brain trust doctors.

One lesson that he learned demonstrates the power of goals.

I told you he had this big goal of going from $5M to $15M, and it was a three-year goal.

At the end of two years, everybody could see that they could coast to get to that by the end of that third year. There was no goal that was compelling because they knew they could get there without even trying.

Guess what happened for the first time in the practice's history?

It went flat.

It had been growing, growing, growing, growing, growing... Great goal. Great vision. But the goal was no longer compelling.

A **compelling goal** is important.

I challenge people when they make their three-year goals. If they understand clearly how they're going to achieve the goal, the goal isn't big enough. It's too tame. It's too low to activate and motivate.

These are the best practices that I've seen when it comes to goal setting and vision.

Why Are You Working Harder and Making Less Money?

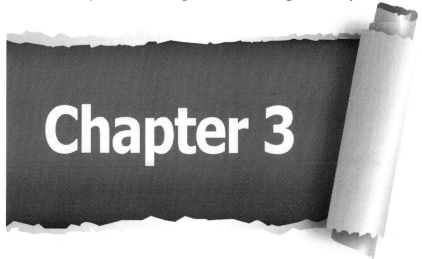

Why Successful Practices are Team Oriented

Habit #2: Become Team Oriented

When I look at the <u>very successful practices... they are team oriented</u>. The way I like to describe it is they worked very hard to find a way that everybody got a piece of what they wanted. It is a win-win-win. This isn't a new concept by any means. Yet it's so rare to see it being done well.

Before I introduce a concept of mental energy, I have a question for you: *"What do you run out of in dentistry first, mental or physical energy?"*

Most people know their answer right away.

In dentistry, we run out of mental energy first. No doubt about it. The successful doctors and practices understand that they have to save every ounce of mental energy because it is a limited resource and is only replenished at a fixed rate.

There's nothing that I'm aware of that speeds replenishment. Therefore, we must be thoughtful about how quickly we drain that energy.

I know teams who will complain about their doctors, saying they have run into their offices and are ignoring everything that's trying to get them back into seeing patients. They'll just sit in their private office.

The reason why we do that is that we are out of mental energy. We burned it all off, and now we've got to let it replenish, and it doesn't replenish quickly; remember, there's no way to make it replenish any faster. Saving every ounce of mental energy is really important.

The Energy Usage Rule

I want to talk about the Energy Usage Rule, and then I'm going to go back to win-win-win. The Energy Usage Rule, and this is important... The way to look at this is to decide how much you'd like to earn each month, then determine how many hours you'd like to work.

We're going to take those earnings, we're going to divide by the hours, and we're going to create our **set point.**

Let's say a dentist wanted to earn a take-home pay of $30,000 per month and they're going to work 120 hours each month.

Divide $30,000 by 120 hours, and you'll come up with $250 per hour. They have to do $250-an-hour work. If they don't do $250-an-hour work, they will not reach their goal.

The Energy Usage Rule is this: Once you've got your set point, any work at the office or at home you can pay someone less than $250 an hour gets hired out.

This was a very difficult thing for me to learn. I'm going to tell you about an embarrassing story of my past. I was a never a 40-hour workweek guy when I was seeing patients. I would work a 10-hour day, come home, have a little dinner, and I'd start working again at night. I did all the accounting: I paid all the bills, I did the payroll, I did the budgeting, I did all the financial reporting, I did it all myself. I also did all the marketing.

I want you to think about how smart that was or wasn't.

I was supposed to be doing $250 an hour, so why was I doing $12-an-hour work? It made no sense at all. <u>It was burning metal energy</u> that I was going to need the next day. This is the Energy Usage Rule. **Don't do any work that you could hire someone else to do for less than your set point.**

You may ask, what constitutes work? Depends on the person. For instance, I had at the time a house with a gigantic yard and large hedges. To mow that yard and do the trimming would take a full day. In the hot summer in Iowa, I'd have to do it at least once a week. I detested that day.

Once a week, I was spending a full day doing yard work. I had a neighbor with the exact same setup. It took him a day, sometimes two. I hated yard work; I absolutely hated it. I mowed lawns for money when I was nine years old and worked it for nine years. I didn't like it then and still don't like it now.

To me, spending that time doing the yard, that was work. My next-door neighbor loved doing yard work. He would be out there in the yard with a mower and be happy as a clam.

Which of us was burning more mental energy? Obviously, it was me. For me, it was work. For him, it was leisure; it was his hobby and he enjoyed it. It depleted my mental energy, but it replenished his.

I had difficulty when I applied this principle into my practice. There were aspects of the practice that I really enjoyed being involved with and others I enjoy personally doing.

I enjoyed budgeting, forecasting, spreadsheets... the numbers piece of it.

If I was going to be maximally productive, I needed to conserve my mentally energy.

If I had chosen to continue to do it, I wouldn't have been able to produce as much. I wouldn't have earned as much. My team wouldn't have earned as much. The entrepreneur gets to choose his or her own vision. He or she also is responsible for the results.

When I started to understand this, I had to make some really big changes. I really enjoyed marketing. I enjoyed learning about it. I enjoyed designing stuff. It would still work and still be draining my mental energy, but I can hire a marketer for $15 an hour. I can't hire somebody for $15 an hour to produce dentistry.

I hired a marketing person.

How you define work is up to you. If it's something that you enjoy and it replenishes and rejuvenates you, keep doing it. Delegate or outsource any work that you can hire someone else to do for less than your set point.

The Delegation Wheel

I see people on the practice treadmill: running, running, running, running, running, running, running, running. They "don't have time to do anything more." They can't grow; they're topped out. Invariably they're failing to delegate effectively.

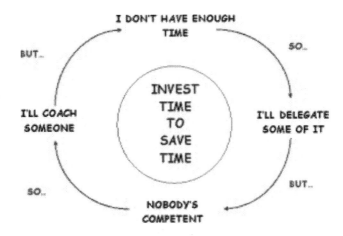

Here's the logic that goes on. "I don't have enough time to do everything I need to do." Then they think, "Okay. I'll delegate some of it." They go to delegate it, but nobody is competent because nobody has been trained.

So then they think…."I'll coach somebody," but I don't have time to coach anybody, and it will be faster if I just do it myself. We're going around the delegation wheel." When it comes to delegation, you really do have to <u>invest time to save time</u>.

I love this quote by Abraham Lincoln. "If I had six hours to chop down a tree, I'd spend the first four hours sharpening the axe." Training your team is like sharpening the axe. The most successful practices are spending <u>several hours a week</u> training team members.

They want everybody to be on board, on task, and ready to perform at an extremely high level. Most practices do not spend nearly enough time training team members. Most practices focus on training forgetting that experienced team members can improve with training too. Most practices don't spend nearly enough time and they would be far more productive in the future.

Teamwork

All of the highly productive practices have another thing in common, they all have a team leader. Some call this person an office manager or a clinic administrator. I'm going to put the word team leader in for our purposes here. The team leader is absolutely a necessity.

The Team Leader Basics...

Doctor runs his clinical schedule, and team leader runs everything else. I've seen many try to implement this and fail.

Why? **It's very common for dentists to give team members the responsibility but not give any authority**. Read that sentence one more time. They give team members responsibility, but they don't give the authority to go with that responsibility.

However, what I find more often than not is they have a title and maybe some responsibility, but they don't have the authority, and they don't have the accountability.

Here's the lessons that I've learned about having a team leader and clinic administrator and my role with that person.

The team leader in my practice, Heather Driscoll, now oversees the operations of about 120 practices in the United States, so she's gone on to great things.

When I started working with her and she was developing in this role and I was developing in maximizing the relationship that she and I had, what I would do is I would tell her what I wanted done.

I would say, "Do this. Do this. Do this. Do this. Do this. These are the steps. Do it this way, this way, this way."

I quickly found that was not very developmental to her.

If we want to advance this position, they have to learn judgment. They have to learn how to think because you're going to be producing. They're going to be making decisions.

So I moved away from talking about "how." I got out of the "how" game completely.

I learned to tell her, "This is the result that I want to see, and I want to see it by this time."

That's all I had to say. She could figure out.

She's, frankly, smarter than I am, so she could figure out how to get there.

Occasionally, she started going in the direction that I could see that there was a pitfall, and so then I had to say something like, "Have you thought about what would happen if this happened?"

She'd go, "Oh, yes. That's not going to work," and she'd adjust and adapt quickly. But I got out of the "how" business.

Once you've identified the ideal result, the team leader's job is to make it happen, and they need to be able to make decisions, and you have to support their decisions even if it's not the same decision that you would make, as long as it's getting to the ideal result. That's what matters.

In a single-doctor practice, this is what I mean by "responsibility" and "authority." "Responsibility" means that they have the ability to make decisions; "authority" means that they are empowered to act on their decisions **without** having to check in and ask for permission for everything.

In my practice, Heather had a $20,000 limit, and if she had to make a decision that involved more than $20,000, she had to talk to me before she did it. Up to $20,000, she could go, she could run with it. Now, that's responsibility and that's authority.

Here's another example where the team leader is running the business. I've observed in many practices dynamic that develops that's extremely unhealthy to the entire practice. It happens when one or two employees start to feel that the rules of the practice do not apply to them. The two people that are most likely to be the culprits of this are also most likely to be the closest to you. This dynamic is more prevalent than you think. It completely undermines your ability to create a team-oriented practice.

Here's what usually happens ... one or two people in the practice will feel like the rules don't apply to them, that they can come and go when they please, they can do the work they want, they can choose to not do the things they don't want to do, and none of the rules including: where to park, where to put your coat, where to put your purse, when you leave for lunch, etc.

Here's how you give authority to your team leader, especially in this situation... The team leader has to have the authority to fire <u>anybody</u>. Anybody who doesn't follow the rules gets progressive coaching up to and including termination. It doesn't matter whether it's the doctor's spouse or whether it is your favorite assistant – your team leader runs the business.

I've seen doctors choose a leader without really understanding WHO should be a team leader. Often, they will choose the person in the office that gets everything done, a "super doer." That is typical and not a bad thing... at first. When you choose someone like that then the doctor does only the things a doctor can do. There's a very interesting lesson with this.

Let's look at corporate dentistry for a moment and look at the incomes of those dentists. They are usually higher than the private practice dentists. Why? Because they don't have to deal with any of the business stuff -- they are solely focused on treating patients and treating patients at a high level. They don't have all the distraction and mental energy burn.

Having a team leader allows a dentist to do only the things that they can do. Only those things that are above their set point.

Here's what so often happens. The doctor says, "I would like you to be more self-reliant, show more initiative, and take greater responsibility, but check with me first."

That's not authority; that's not responsibility. That's not what I'm talking about. I'm talking about, let them run. Now, are they going to make mistakes? Absolutely. Are they going to make big mistakes? Absolutely.

But they have to learn somehow. You get started and you give them **guidance**, **you ask them questions**, but you want them to **develop** the judgment to make good decisions. Good judgment comes from experience.

Mistakes and Perfection

When you start this process, your team leader will make mistakes.

Just like you would.

But here is the interesting thing.

What I have found when I do a project or something and it's all done and I look back at it, I would learn some stuff during the process.

I would say, "That's pretty good. I'm glad it's done, but if I had to do it over again, I would have done this or this or this differently."

When I get all done and I'm very proud and I look back on it, it's about 80% of the way to being perfect. 20% I would do differently. 80% of the way to being perfect is fine.

But here's what happens. When you begin to delegate things, other people are going to take it over. You know what they're going to do? They're going to get it about 80% right.

Here's the problem that gets us stuck. The 20% that didn't go right for the team leader is going to be a different 20% that didn't go right if you did it.

What do we do? We automatically judge their 20%. We think it's an obvious mistake. We lose confidence.

That's what traps us.

We should be saying, "Okay. We got 20% that wasn't perfect. Very good. 80% of it that's right. It's done. Great. Let's move on."

Don't expect perfection. People are going to make mistakes.

The only way that you can max out as a dentist is by doing only those things that dentist can do.

Let's go back to WHO we should choose as the team leader. When we choose the person in the office who always gets everything done, there is one big issue that will pop up…. They will tend to micromanage everything.

Micromanagement Avoidance Formula

The Micromanagement Avoidance Formula is simple. Create a clear and concise vision of what the desired completed project looks like, so we have a clear "what."

Create a clear timeline, ensuring only one person is responsible. Avoid the "how." Once you get into the "how" you are micromanaging. When people understand what they're supposed to accomplish and they understand when they have to get it done, they'll figure out how. They'll figure out how, and they'll have a lot more fun figuring out the how and doing it their own way rather than having someone tell them step-by-step or exactly what to do. Stay away from the how. Often, the super doers will have a very difficult time staying away from the how. This can lead to the "best is your worst" syndrome.

The Best Is Your Worst Syndrome

Often, that person who is the super doer, who takes everything on, who gets everything done, who's very consistent, very high energy, very positive attitude, they'll take everything on to the point where they get full. Once that person gets full of the practices trapped, they can't grow because the obstacle to doing more is that person.

Your very best person can often can be the person that's holding you back from growth. They don't know it, and you don't know it. You only know that you are stuck, but you don't know why.

At one of our Blue Diamond retreats (with our high-level coaching clients), we experienced this firsthand with a practice who couldn't figure why they had stopped growing. They were stuck because of the "best is your worst syndrome."

Ultimately, it came down to the fact that they had a great Team Leader who was willing to work hard, willing to do everything, but she was full. She had never trained anybody to do what she does, never delegated. She never let people try and fail. She never let them have that authority AND responsibility of doing their jobs on their own.

She was the blockage. She was bright; she was hardworking, she was passionate; she was super. But she was also the worst thing happening in their practice because she was holding it back. Watch out for the your-best-is-your-worst syndrome; it sneaks up.

So who should be a team leader?

Identifying Leaders

People tell me, "I don't have any leaders or potential leaders in my practice."

I tell them, baloney. You may not have someone identified, someone with the title, but you've got a leader. I can tell you; there is someone that's leading your practice that maybe you aren't aware of, but they are.

I have used exercises in the past to help identify the leader. They usually consisted of putting the group in certain situations and watching who people follow.

I know practices that have done things like obstacle courses, and just by observing, you will see somome exhibit leadership.

My partner, Wendy Briggs, discovered an excellent example of this while attending a mastermind group in the UK, where someone shared a really interesting interview process that revolutionized finding team members that fit.

One of the things that was really interesting is they had all the candidates who'd passed the initial phone interview, who passed muster with the team, come at exactly the same time.

You have, say, four top candidates for an administrative position at the front desk. They had them all come at the same time, and they did group interviews.

One of the things they did while they all were there together is they gave them a task.

They gave them a stack of books and DVDs and video cases and things, and they put the stack in the center of the room.

They said, "Okay. Here's your challenge. You have three minutes to build a tower that's a certain height and that can hold a cup of water."

Then they stepped back and they watched.

Each observer team member was assigned to look for certain characteristics that would shine through. What they discovered was that, in this exercise, naturally, there was someone who would take charge.

They're looking for "Do they play well with others? Are they patient? Are they helpful or are they sharp or snapping at the people that they're trying to work with? Did they engage the other candidates in a solution? Did they include everyone? Did people follow their lead?"

They were identifying what characteristics they could see from them having to do this task together.

The results are really interesting. All the candidates want to look the best because they're vying for this job. They discovered almost everyone is impressed by the same individual.

There is one person that will shine through that task that is impressive.

They've got it down to almost a science now that, within a minute of the task beginning, they know who they're going to hire. They know who the best fit is for their team.

You can see how you could design something like that for your office team and see how they function together. This is yet another example of team involvement.

Team Involvement

Team involvement is important. People support what they help create. The observer team members are invested in the success of the candidate chosen because they were a part of the decision.

Use this same tactic when you have a project that needs to be done. And don't plan it out to the nth degree. As a leader, identify what the ideal result is. Throw it out to the team:

- What do you guys think?

- How are we going to do this?

Then stay quiet.

If they figure out how to do it, now they're invested. Now they have ownership in that project. They have ownership in its success. And if it fails, they're a part of it too.

Planning

Many of us are planners. We think things through. "Okay. We're going to now bring implant dentistry into our practice. The first thing we're going to do is this, and the next thing that we're going to do is this, and the next thing we're going to do is this."

We get it all planned out, and then you tell your teams what to do.

For many of us, that's our natural leadership style. Certainly, it was mine.

I wasn't sure I could do it, particularly, early on.

I would create a project. I would go through this entire planning process, but I wouldn't show my results to the team.

I would tell the team, "Here's the ideal result. How are you going to get there?" I already had it thought through, but I led the team to think through it together. You know what happened? They would develop plans. If I saw them going in a direction that I thought wouldn't work, I would ask them a question. "That sounds good, but what would happen if ..." that would highlight the pitfall that I saw.

When I got good at doing it, I found that they found a way to get to that result. I didn't need to say much. I didn't need to ask many questions.

I was surprised that they developed a plan that was often better than mine.

They are seeing the practice from a different perspective, and so they see pitfalls that I could never have seen. We end up with a better result.

Standards

The next thing about team involvement is important and counterintuitive.

Team members are craving standards.

When there are no standards there, they feel lost.

Do they like standards all the time? No.

"Here's our dress code. This is how you are to look when you come in the office." That's a standard. That gives confidence to people. They know they're doing good.

When there's a standard and they're living up to that standard, they know they're doing well. That's very comforting for team members.

Now, when don't they like it?

When they have to be held accountable. Most don't like that part.

The reason why we are so standard-less in dentistry is the only feedback we give is negative, when you're holding them accountable.

I can tell you, when I meet with teams and their doctor is not in the room, they tell me over and over again, "*We don't know what we're supposed to do.*"

They are craving for standards. Don't expect them to appreciate it.

The bottom line is that the only way for true growth is to become a team-oriented practice. In order to do this, you need to:

- Know your set point

- Correctly delegate to your team

- Identify a team leader who has responsibility, accountability, and authority in your practice

- Train your team and your team leader

- Know that they will make mistakes and it is from these mistakes that your team will grow

- Set standards and hold people accountable for them

Why Are You Working Harder and Making Less Money?

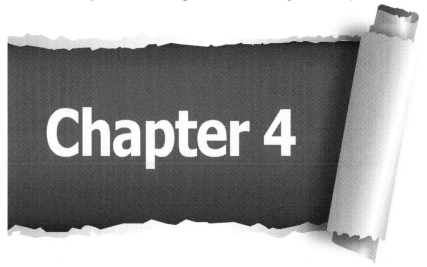

The Difference Between Good and Great

Habit #3: Instill Discipline

Highly effective practices have a level of discipline that I did not notice in the people that were just focusing on being clinicians.

I'm going to pick just a handful of the disciplines that I noticed in these superstars:

- Stick to the Vision and Goals
- Meetings
- Follow the Rules

Shiny Object Syndrome

The first thing to sticking to your vision and goals is to control the *shiny object syndrome*. This syndrome is very common among dentists in general. Particularly among these very high-performing folks. I think each of them being entrepreneurs willing to risk, willing to grow, willing to move things, willing to make something big happen, all of them had, I believe, a little touch of ADD. Part of their struggle was to stay focused.

So how did they do it? There are three key ways I found.

1. **Quarterly planning process**. This is 90-day discipline. You create your plan for the next 90 days, and you don't deviate from the plan. 90 days later you can make a new plan. Anything that you learn or anything that you notice or anything that you want to do within that 90-day period needs to wait for the start of the next 90-day period. That way, you focus only on the things that are on your plan and don't get distracted by other things. I have seen so many dentists spend so much money learning this or that only to go and have something else catch their attention. Now they're off learning that without ever having implemented the first things that they learned. Very, very, very, very common. That's why this

quarterly planning process is important to stay focused on the things that matter.

2. **Have a key team member**. If you don't have one of these, I hope you search for one and find one. That's the team member who's bold enough to tell you the truth whether you want to hear it or not. They're the ones who call you out when you misbehave, when you don't follow agreements, and when you make mistakes. I was very fortunate to have several team members who would call me out when I needed it. It can be hard. Everybody wants to hear that they're great all the time, but sometimes the dynamics in a dental office are such that, the dentist doesn't get the brutral feedback when they need it. The dentist needs to know when there are things that they can improve upon significantly.

3. **A personal board of directors**. I've been fortunate to have built a very elaborate set of directors, and I've spent a lot of time developing this group. My group consists of my personal finance mentor, my personal business strategist, an attorney, an ex-CEO, and several highly successful entrepreneurs. I have both dentists and non-dentists on my personal board. But they are all people that I admire and who live their lives the way I want to live my life. You want to find

mentors whom you aspire to be like. It is far easier to copy genius than to create mediocrity.

When I have a question, when I'm feeling overwhelmed, when I feel like I'm losing my focus, I can call one of these guys or gals up and take them out for coffee or out for lunch. Most of them don't know each other, we don't meet in a group, but I go to them with specific things when I need help, guidance, or motivation.

Having a personal board of directors is very helpful. For members of The Team Training Institute, this is one of the roles we play -- we help doctors and team members network with other practices so that they create their own board of directors.

These are the people that you can call to keep you on track and help you avoid becoming distracted by the latest greatest gadget, the best salesman, the shiny object that promises to solve all of your problems.

Shiny object syndrome is a very common trait in dentists. The problem is, there will never be 'one thing' to solve every problem. I wish there were, but there just isn't one thing. To grow successfully, you have to solve a lot of problems and do a lot of things right to be successful.

The first discipline: avoiding shiny object syndrome.

Great Meetings

The next discipline is having great meetings. I have seen some great successful meetings and I've seen some terrible failures. Here is the meeting structure that I've seen work in practices that are successful at improving their performance.

Morning Huddles: The first one is a **morning huddle**. I have seen good morning huddles that were informational, educational, and inspiring. I've seen huddles where people leave fired up to greet the day. I've also seen huddles where the walking dead leave the huddle to under-inspire their patients and teammates.

Morning huddles are a must for practices that are successfully engaging people to maximize patient service and the patient experience.

I break the morning huddle down into two pieces.

First is results. How did we do yesterday? Are we on track?

Second is how do we make today the best it can be?

I like to start a morning huddle with a quick review of the numbers from the previous day, celebrating anything that stands out. Keyword there: CELEBRATING.

If somebody had a bad day, we don't even mention it. The purpose of the huddle is to increase everybody's confidence, not to beat anybody down. These are <u>meetings</u>, not beatings!

Then I look on the schedule for opportunities.

This is done differently depending on the size of your practice. If you've got six doctors in the same location who are all starting at the same time, you can't go through each and every schedule and look for opportunities with the entire team. It would simply take too much time and cover too much information that would not directly affect everyone.

What I'm describing for you is the huddle of a single-doctor and maybe two-doctor practice.

As well as looking for opportunities that day, you want to cover any personal information about the patients that not everybody knows – like "Sally got married last week; Mary's husband died since the last time she was here," those kinds of things.

Then included in 'opportunities' are people on the doctor's schedule that are due in hygiene and people in hygiene that have diagnosed and undone treatment. Because you're trying to prepare to deliver these services while the patient is there…that day!

Then the last part of the morning huddle is some type of educational and energy piece.

One option is to create a weekly schedule. It doesn't need to be this methodical but you'll get the picture:

- Mondays: People bring in a favorite funny YouTube video.

- Tuesdays: We would do an educational game. For instance, we liked the grab the marker game. We'd put a marker in the middle of our conference table, and I would ask a dental diagnosis or treatment-related question. The first person who grabbed it and could answer the question would win a prize.

- Wednesdays: Food. So we always had some healthy treats on Wednesdays.

- Thursdays: A game just for fun. Sometimes a Minute to Win It. You can go on YouTube and find Minute to Win It videos and directions. Most are very easy and funny. That require very minimal setup.

- Sometimes we would throw up a dental case. We'd pick someone at random to do the treatment plan. It could be anybody. It could be an assistant; it could be the front office person. If the janitor was walking through, we'd grab him, put him in there. It could be anybody.

The point is you discuss cases and people do the treatment planning even if they aren't treatment planners. Their level of understanding of what you would do starts to improve, their judgment improves, and their ability to talk and communicate about it improves.

All these things just fire people up and get people ready to greet the day.

The idea is that when people leave the morning huddle, they should have the attitude that they're going to have the most amazing day.

The leader's role for a morning huddle is to manage the energy and the attitude of the people. You're giving information, doing some educational piece, providing some connection between the team and patients, and providing some cohesion between the team.

Why have I seen so many terrible failures when it comes to morning huddles? Because the doctor isn't willing to set the boundaries and enforce the rules. Here are some simple morning huddle rules.

1. Everybody must be there. Including, and especially, the doctor. It is mandatory for everyone on the team to be there.

2. Everybody must be prepared. Everyone brings something to the meeting. If you're a clinical team member, you're bringing a schedule. What are you seeing for opportunities in your schedule? If you're an administrative team member, you're bringing stats, you're bringing information on new patients that will be seen today, and you're bringing information on people that are possibilities for same-day treatment opportunities.

The morning huddle takes place every morning. I found that this entire meeting can be accomplished in just 15 minutes <u>even if</u> you have a relatively big practice.

You spend the first 10 minutes going through the stats from yesterday, new patients being seen today, and same-day dentistry opportunities. The next five minutes are spent getting the entire team pumped up and ready for the day.

The leader's goal for the morning huddle is that everyone is informed and ready for the day.

People rarely get pumped up if they don't move. Getting people to move, to stand up, to do high-fives, to watch somebody do a Minute to Win It …everybody up and moving is how people start the day with a lot of energy.

I can tell you, if you watch really successful people in any field, they start strong, right? They start strong; they start together. Great bands, they start together. Great athletes, they start together.

Think about track and field sprint races, they're over at the start. If you get a bad start, you can't catch up. It's over. Having a very strong start is really important. That's what the morning huddle is designed to do.

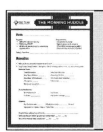

If you would like to download my daily huddle worksheets, they are a part of the free toolkit you can download at:
www.11HabitsToolkit.com

Weekly Team Meetings: The second type of meeting that successful practices conduct is a weekly team meeting. Some practices can get away with bi-weekly meeting but usually monthly is not often enough.

The weekly team meeting consists of a little bit of many things: problem solving, planning, training, connecting, processes, relationships, and results. The weekly team meeting is a check-in on how everybody is doing as a team. It's an opportunity for people to bring up anything they want to discuss, to make an opportunity list and prioritize the list. Every team meeting should have training.

If you find that your meetings start to descend into more of a "gripe session" than a productive meeting, you might want to try this:

Have every single person say one thing that's going right in their personal or professional life.

Our 38 team members went around the room and said one thing that was going right in their personal or professional life.

When you have that much positive momentum, everybody's talking about the good things, good things, good things, good things, good things, good things, it's hard within an hour to degrade into a gripe session. It was very helpful for us.

We call that the Positive Focus.

What Causes Meetings to Fail?

What causes team meetings to fail? Most common reason by far, the person running the meeting is not prepared. These meetings are not something leaders just show up for and facilitate; there needs to be preparation.

The minimum prep is two hours for every hour of meeting. That's the absolute minimum. A team meeting that is dull, disorganized, and doesn't start and end on time shows that someone did not spend an adequate amount of time preparing. Two hours for every hour of meeting. There doesn't have to be a single person doing that two hours, but that's what it takes at a minimum.

Annual Planning Meetings:

The best annual planning meetings are off-site and one day long. You need to get out of your regular grind and really dig in. You want to answer questions like:

- What are we going to accomplish over the next year?

- What are our numeric goals? What numbers are we going to hit?

- What's our revenue goal going to be? How much are doctors going to do? How much will come from hygiene? How much comes from each provider?

- What are all the things that we want to implement?

- What do we want to do to improve our patient experience?

- What do we want to do to improve our marketing and public relations?

- What do we want to do to improve our facility?

- What do we want to do to improve our capabilities?

- What do we want to do to improve our profitability for stability and growth?

All of those questions are answered at that annual planning meeting.

The outcome of this yearly meeting should be clarity on your three-year and one-year goals. You will also set up the first 90-day sprint which describes in detail what will be accomplished by who during the following 90 days. 90 days later you have a quarterly planning meeting where you plan the next 90 days. This is a very disciplined meeting structure. It happens the same way every quarter every year.

Quarterly Planning Meetings:

The quarterly planning meeting is getting the team together and deciding what you're going to accomplish over the next 90 days – and only the next 90 days. It's between 3 and 3 ½ hours long.

These 90-day sprints, as we call them, are a way to really get everybody focused and to provide clarity on who is responsible to do what in the next 90 days. *What is it that we want to accomplish* and *who is going to be responsible for what in 90 days?*

It's important to get the timing of the meeting right; this is what worked for us:

- Morning huddle – 15 minutes tops.

- Weekly or biweekly – an hour and a half.

- Quarterly planning meetings – half day.

- Yearly planning session – one day.

The quarterly and yearly planning meetings were just the leadership: the doctors and team/department leaders. The morning huddles and the weekly meetings include everyone.

The 10-20-70 Rule

Why is it that turnover is so destructive to dental practices? Because with high turnover, you operate with a team that is highly inexperienced and lacking knowledge in your practice. You operate with team members who do not have relationships with your patient base. They may make more mistakes. They may offend people. They don't perform well at this high level, yet. They're not as fast. They're not as intuitive. The only way to get them there is through training and learning.

What we know is that people learn 10% from a lecture format. 20% from being mentored, guided, or coached. And the final 70% comes from doing.

How can you use this 10-20-70 rule to help your practice learn new things? How can you use the 10-20-70 concept in your weekly meetings, your morning huddles to progress your team's learning?

What can we set up so that our teams have a chance to hear, they have a chance to be coached, and their performance monitored and guided and improved?

What do we set up so that they can actually do it? One of the things I love to use is role-playing. With role-playing, people learn so much faster than just listening to a lecture.

I recently set up an experience for a small group of doctors – it was both fascinating and eye opening for the doctors and me. I taught them some concepts related to their initial exam. They then role-played using that new concept.

The smart women and men who now understood the concepts performed poorly. I coached them and then they role-played it again. It was amazing how much faster people got it when we used this technique vs. just listening to a lecture and then being expected to go out and perform.

It's really important to remember that 70% of what we learn comes from doing. You can't just expect to tell someone something once or twice and then expect them to perform well. It takes practice and coaching to improve. The 10-20-70 principle obviously applies to ourselves as well as our teams. How do we get meaningful information, experience, and coaching?

The second discipline: Have a disciplined meeting cadence.

Everyone MUST Follow the Rules

The next discipline is that everybody has to follow the rules. Every practice has rules, processes, procedures, and best practices. Some of the rules are stated. Some of the rules aren't stated. But we know there are rules in every single dental practice.

Who are the worst offenders? Who are the rule breakers in most dental practices? No doubt about it, the doctors are the most likely offenders.

What I found in these really highly performing practices is that the doctors had the attitude that they were a member of the team. They had the "we're a team and we're all in this together and we're all going to follow the rules" attitude. It was a "we are all going to do it together, and nobody is going to be special or different or above the rules" attitude.

When any team member feels that the rules don't apply to them, the team camaraderie is destroyed. Clearly camaraderie is needed to be a highly performing team.

In high-performing teams, everybody follows the rules.

What are the rules I see broken?

1. **On time.** Everybody has to be on time. If you're not on time, then you're not part of the team. If you don't feel like you have to be on time and everybody else does, is that a team? That's drifting more into the family, isn't it? I can tell you, families are great and wonderful and sweet, but they don't necessarily get much done.

2. **Uniform.** Everybody has to be in uniform. However, you define that for your practice. When one or two people don't abide by the uniform rule, the rest of the team feel like those people aren't really a part of the team. The non-conformers think they are above or better than others. People acting this way will destroy cohesion and engagement.

3. **Clean up after yourself.** Another rule I see broken all the time is the "clean up after yourself" rule. I was in a practice just recently and having

lunch with the doctor in the break room. We started to talk to some of his team members. The doctor excused himself. He left his dishes on the table. He went in his office and got on a sports website. I thought, "Okay. Now, somebody has got to clean this up." They clean up their own stuff, but somebody is going to have to clean up after the doctor. This may seem like a little thing, but they aren't little things; they're big things. Because if you're trying to drive a team to get to a very high level of performance, you can't take liberties like this because the team will resent it. When they resent it, the only way they have to get back is to not perform as well as they could. That's the only thing they can do.

4. **Meetings**. I can't tell you how many times teams have huddles with no doctor there. Loses all the punch. Loses all the power. It just isn't worth what it costs you. Follow the rules just like everybody else. Leaders go first on the hard tasks, they eat last, and build the confidence of those around them by being one of them. Quite simply, doctors don't have a choice of whether or not to be a leader. Due to your title and your license you are a leader. Your choice is to be a good one or a bad one.

I have a practice that I have watched for some time. It was a very high-performing practice, and then the practice was sold. The new dentist came in and thought that the rules don't apply to her.

For instance, this was a practice that didn't have adequate parking. All the team parked in the parking lot a block away and they walked (and this was in a northern climate, so there was snow and rain, yucky winter weather). This doctor decided that she was going to park in the patient parking area right by the door.

That one action was incredibly demoralizing to the team. They felt like there was no longer a team, that they weren't all in this together. They felt there is now a queen bee. "All the rest of us have to sludge through the snow and the mud and everything to get to the practice." I had the ability to watch the numbers in this practice. No surprise. They've just drifted down and down and down. High performance doesn't happen without teamwork. Teamwork will not happen if the doctor feels they are above the team.

The third discipline: Follow the rules.

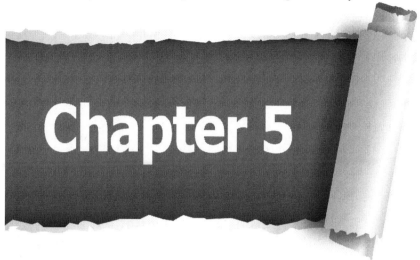

Becoming Service Oriented

Habit #4: Become service oriented

I like to start talking about service by thinking about this as a philosophy of being charitable. That's charitable with the team, with patients, with the community, and with the profession.

Let's start by looking at being charitable with the team. What does this mean? I don't mean just finding ways to hand out lots of extra money... what I mean is that you try and find a way to say "yes." That you create a bias for saying yes vs. saying no.

The same with patients. If they want X, Y, or Z. "Yes, we'll do everything that we can to make that happen for you." This is a 'Yes' bias versus 'No' bias.

Being charitable in the community… this is something that many practices are doing and finding not only personally gratifying but have seen how being charitable in the community grows their practice.

Let's look at a couple of the practices that I studied…

One of the doctors in my mentor group was Dr. Vince Monticciolo. Some of you may have heard of him before. He is the founder of Dentistry From The Heart.

Dentistry From The Heart is an organization that supports dental practices who have a desire to serve their community with a free day of dentistry. You can find many resources for holding a free dental event at: www.dentistryfromtheheart.org. They have resources to help you organize, market, and provide a great experience for these patients and your team.

Dr. Monticciolo told me that his goal was to find a way to support practices to give a million dollars of dentistry. Well, he passed a million dollars years ago. If you just Google "Dentistry From The Heart," you'll see, there are tons of practices all over the United States and Canada that participate in Dentistry From The Heart. It's a great program. I have participated in many of these events and hope to do many more.

Vince was really instrumental in starting this program and bringing awareness to it. He spent at least a year speaking at every dental meeting, every place in the United States he could, in order to build this up, and it's far beyond what he could have ever imagined.

Another office uses the Crime Scene Investigation theme. They had T-shirts made with the same colors and patterns that you would see on the TV show CSI. But instead of saying Crime Scene Investigation, it said Community Service Initiative. At their annual meeting, they committed to do a charitable activity every other month. The team chose to do: Dentistry From The Heart, a separate free day for children (Little Hearts, Big Smiles), ringing the Salvation Army bells, Toys for Tots, and several very clever charitable activities.

They did a children's Halloween-themed safety event for the community. They set up a little street fair, and they invited the police, fire department, and other emergency personnel to come and do safety training for the kids. The kids would climb on the fire truck, hop in the ambulance, and sit in a police car. The kids would come in their costumes and learn fun safety techniques.

These things are all great for the community. All of them received some media coverage and some PR benefit from it. But I don't think that's what the major benefit was. The **major benefit is the team doing things together** in service of others. It's such a great team-building experience. It is such a culture builder to do these kinds of events. The real value comes from the connections, relationships, and the bond that they create together as a team.

That's what I mean when I talk about a charitable philosophy. Everyone gives their time, their talent, and their treasure to their patients and the community around them.

What Do Patients Want?

Another way to be charitable is to focus on what your current patients want. Zig Ziglar has a statement that I love and I believe is fundamental:

"You can get everything you want in life if you just help enough other people get what they want."

I speak all over the United States and Canada for different kinds of groups, and there is an exercise I often do. It's fascinating to me because I go to a flip chart and I say, "What do patients want?"

The dentist and their teams in the audience say things like:

- Quality care

- Attractive dentistry

- Painless

Yes, we all want quality care. We all want to have beautiful restorations. We all want it to be painless.

Then we get to the things that we know patients want but it's not what we want. Do patients want to wait? Not many do. Most patients want what they want and they want it now.

Do we want them to wait? Not really but if they have to wait, they have to wait, right?

Do patients want you to take their insurance? Yes. We prefer our full fee.

Do patients want convenient hours? Yes. But convenient hours for most patients is when they're not working – which means evenings, early mornings, noon, weekends.

How do we feel about those hours? Not so great, right?

Do patients like to be referred out to another office? No, they don't.

Some dentists don't like to treat children, do oral surgery, do endo, etc.

We know what patients want, we really do. You could do this exercise with your team and find similar results. Ask your team what patients want and make a list.

I would advise you to lead your team to pick one or two things on that list to implement. Move just one step closer to what your patients want.

It doesn't have to be earth-shattering. It doesn't have to be amazing, but if you regularly do this exercise and move one step, over time your practice will become more and more patient friendly.

Now, why is being patient friendly so important?

You've read the study, right? If somebody comes to your office and has a bad experience, how many people will they tell? Six or seven? If they have a good experience, they'll tell how many? One, right?

Wrong! That's completely wrong. That's how it used to be.

Today, with a few keystrokes, press enter, they can tell thousands of people.

Do you know how I know this? One of the practices I am working with has a very bad Google review. There's probably not a lot of truth in the Google review but probably enough truth to know that it was a bad experience. The review has 13,000 views. The town the practice serves only has 7,000 people in it.

Today we've got to be really, really good operationally because people are choosing their practitioners based on their online reputations. These reviews matter. Your rankings matter. Give patients what they want, be amazing, and your reviews will reflect it.

Can't Give Good Away

Another service principle I learned from my mentor, Vince Zirpoli.

His exact quote is:

"You can't give good away because it comes back 10 times to you."

One way of applying the principle is to think about doing the extra for your patient.

Every dental team has a habitual way of treating patients. There's a certain way you do things. What if you think each day, "How can I do a little bit extra?"

- Maybe it's a little bit more time.

- Maybe it's a little bit more compassion.

- Maybe it's a little more interest in the person as a person.

If you can do a little bit better, that good will come back to you 10 times over.

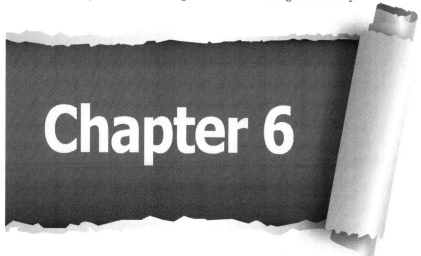

How Do You Know You're Doing Well?

Habit #5: Know Your Statistics

I'm going to let you in on something. I have always said that within about 20 seconds of being in an office, I can get a very, very good feel on how well that practice is doing. It is almost instantaneous when you know what to look for.

While touring any practice (and finding something to compliment them on), I will say, "I like the way you do this... How is the practice doing?" Generally, I'll get an answer like, "Oh, things are going just great." To which I then ask, "How do you know?"

That's the trick ... how do you know? The answer to that question will tell you a lot about a person's capabilities.

If they say "Well, we're up this year 15% over last year. Our profitability is up 20%. Our new patient numbers are growing. Even better yet, our case acceptance is up."

That's an answer from somebody who knows their business. Occasionally, they'll have no answer at all. Sometimes the answer goes something like this, "Well, everybody's getting along pretty good." Which tells you what the standard is which they use to judge their success. Every really well-run hyper productive practice is following their statistics.

Consider this … You want to be looking at numbers that are helpful in measuring how well you're doing and can help you make decisions about how you could do better. This includes current numbers, past numbers and the trends that they make plus ratios.

Here is what I like to look at:

** Profitability: You have to understand your practice's profitability.

I recently met a manager who was managing two relatively big practices. The owner of the practices wouldn't let her see the financial information about the practice. She had no idea whether she was running a profitable business or a non-profitable business … no idea.

So was she really running it?

No, because she didn't have the information that she needed to make good decisions about how to improve the practice.

I recently looked at a practice to acquire. They were doing about $5 million in revenue. Sounds like a great practice, right?

Then I ask the big one. "Well, that's $5 million. That's great. How profitable are you?" Well, it turns out this practice was losing money which is why it was for sale. They were bringing in a lot of money, but they were spending even more. Profitability, that's a very, very important number to follow.

** **Internal referrals.** This will tell you how well your patients like the experience that they are receiving in your practice. If they're happy with what happens in your office, they're going to be glad to tell their friends and family. If they aren't happy with the experience, then your referral number will be low. If your service is worsening or is not keeping up with your competitors, your referrals will shrink and shrink and shrink.

I have a practice that I'm watching implode right now that is really a very, very sad situation. He's a doctor in a small town, and his practice style is certainly not patient centric, not patient comfort centric. It's not physically or emotionally comfortable.

He is a gruff and rude and kind of rough in his treatment. He doesn't connect with people well. Now his social media profile is unbelievably bad. His new patient flow is drying up. His practice is in a death spiral.

I'm trying to help him get out of it, but he just doesn't understand that internal referrals are a key number. <u>If you don't have 50% of your new patients coming from patient referrals, you have a patient experience problem</u>.

If I only had two numbers that I could track in an office to make decisions about what to do, the first one would be the big one and that's profitability; the second would be internal referrals. Here are a few more that I do look at:

1. **Production and Collections.** If you look at production this year versus last year, that gives you the past and the current. Therefore, you can see the trend. Then same with collections. Then if you compare collections to production -- so you get your collections percentage -- that would be a ratio.

2. **Expenses**. Ideally, we have those expenses broken down into different categories so that we

can see how we're doing. You may have budgeted 25% of revenue to pay for salaries, not including doctors. Comparing what you actually spent to what you planned to spend is very helpful.

3. **New patients.** Important to know this number and to know what the trend is. If the trend of new patients is going down, if you have any chance of growing the practice, your case acceptance has to be going up. Declining number of new patients is not necessarily a bad thing if you're able to do more on the patients that you're getting.

4. **Accounts receivable**. I had a client that we worked with that had raised their productivity by a million dollars in one year. They almost doubled their production in one year. The doctor called and said, "Well, this really stinks because I'm not making any more money." I said, "It would be impossible to double your production and not make a whole lot more money." But as it turned out, they <u>weren't collecting</u> any of it.

They weren't even trying to collect any of it. Their accounts receivable had grown dramatically and he had no idea because he wasn't watching the production/collection ratio and he wasn't watching his accounts receivable number.

By the time I figured this out for him, he was fairly far down the road that some of these account balances were so old, he was never going to collect them.

5. **Insurance AR.** What do you have out in insurance claims? If you're taking insurance, you have to watch, what are they paying? When are they paying? How long is it taking?

6. **Hygiene Numbers**. There are a few things from hygiene that we need to keep an eye on.

    a. Case Acceptance from hygiene

    b. Perio. As a percentage of hygiene and a percentage of the total practice.

7. **Patient retention**

8. **Team retention**

9. **Marketing expenses**

10. **Missed and cancelled appointments**

11. **Hours worked**

Tracking

Based on these numbers, you can compare numbers using ratios. For example, Case Average is a ratio between collections and new patients.

We had the most amazing thing happen to one of our clients. We were tracking his numbers and noticed a huge gain in productivity.

He was at the time of his yearly review with his Team Training Institute admin coach and he says, "We're so much more productive. I'm so proud. We're up 25%, but I'm a little disappointed that we didn't make any more money." Huh?

How do you produce 25% more and not end up with any more profit?

There's two ways:

1. You spent too much.

2. You were producing it but not collecting it.

So he was so proud of his production, and he should be because that was a lot of good work. To go up 25% in production, you have to make significant changes. In an established mature practice, change is hard.

25% is a big gain! In his case his team discontinued following the practice's financial arrangement process. Any practice could increase production 25% if they didn't have to collect it. So watching the accounts receivable is really important.

Keep It Simple

I have seen practices that create a report every month, print it out, and it's a thick document.

There was a lot of great information in there, but it was so much that nobody could watch it and, more importantly, nobody could follow it. Therefore, it was not a useful tool for driving change.

I like to keep things simple. Focused information is more powerful.

If you're trying to create change, focus the numbers you are reporting to just a few including numbers that relate to the change you are trying to create.

Let's use our client whose production went up but collections did not. We recommended that he retrain on the financial arrangement process that had been successful in the past. Next, we focused the numbers that were reported daily at their morning huddle. We chose one number to report: percentage of daily production that was collected over the counter.

This number went from 7% to 40% in just a few weeks. Productivity suffered slightly, but total collections improved and profitability soared.

To be an effective manager, you need to analyze your performance. Next, identify where you need to improve. Determine that data that will allow you to measure short-term and long-term progress. Report the results to the team so they can feel their progress. If they are not making progress, it is likely there is a problem with either the process (95% of the time) or the people (5%).

Why Are You Working Harder and Making Less Money?

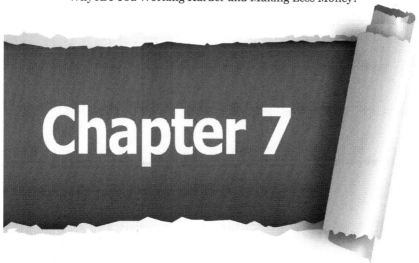

Help! We've Plateaued

Habit #6: Be aware of capacity

If your practice is not growing, there are only two possible reasons why. The big one (and the one that most people don't see) is that the practice is out of capacity. The other reason is that you have a patient experience problem. Most people are walking around with blinders on, unable to see either issue.

Most people believe that if you want your practice to grow simply, do more marketing. That is just not quite true – because if you don't have a good patient experience or you are out of capacity and you do a lot of marketing, you will actually drive your practice down.

You will be bringing in a lot of people to then go spread the word around about the crappy experience they had. Or worse yet, drive people to call your practice to only find out that they can't get an appointment. Marketing will speed up practice growth or practice decline, but it won't change the direction.

Here's my personal experience with a capacity blockage. I had a consultant come into my office, and he looked around.

He said, "You're out of treatment rooms. You need more ops."

Where I was standing when he told me this, I could see, in the middle of the day, three empty ops.

So what did I do?

I argued with him.

I didn't believe him because, in my perspective, I was seeing the three empty ops. I wasn't seeing the schedule that was getting booked out further and further. I had blinders on.

We argued for a while, and finally, he said, "How much are you collecting? How many ops do you have?"

He did a little math, and he said, "Okay. You're doing $20,000 per op per month, so you need three more ops."

I argued with that, and he was getting mad. Finally, he said, "$60,000 a month, that's what you're losing here."

Before he left, I got on the phone with the contractor and an architect. We put three ops in.

Within four months, we were up $60,000 a month.

We were blocked, and I couldn't see it.

What is Capacity?

Because it's not just ops. Some of the elements that contribute to your capacity are:

- Treatment rooms
- Equipment
- Supplies
- Number of employees
- Number of parking spots
- Systems
- Team member engagement
- Doctor's level of engagement

If you don't have these in the right ratios, you're going to experience capacity problems.

How do you spot when you have a capacity problem?

They are very, very difficult to spot. I like to say people have blinders on when it comes to capacity. They really do.

What are some of the capacity issues that I've seen?

On the **people** side, not enough assistants. That's very common.

In most practices, you can find the minimum number of assistants. Take the number of rooms you have minus the number of hygienists you have. That's a minimum number.

We're talking about full time equivalents, assuming you're not working a split schedule.

Another people blockage that we see frequently is not enough people at the front desk to enable good financial arrangements to be made.

If we don't have someone that can help a patient walk through each of the financial options, including a third-party finance application, we don't have enough people.

The **places** that we run out of most often is ops. There are no quick, easy, and inexpensive options to fix this issue.

Another place that you can run out of is no private place to talk about money with patients; that's a place that's commonly missing.

Things that are missing. For example, not having treatment rooms equally equipped; having that one treatment room that doesn't get used very often and nobody wants to use it because it's got crappy stuff in it. Getting all of the materials and equipment for the team to work efficiently is a key to improved productivity.

Systems. Most of the time, practices start growing, they become successful because of the people. But if you're dependent on people and that person leaves, you're in trouble.

Smaller practices tend to not have systems as they grow.

You start having difficulty because the next person coming in may not be as talented as the one that you just had and now you've got a problem.

So we should be building practices on systems, in addition to great people.

Time. Usually it's doctor's time. The ideal is a doctor who is moving steadily from patient to patient doing treatment and exams throughout the day. Never rushed … never slowing down. The reality is a patient comes late, a procedure takes longer than expected, hygiene exams back up, etc. Each of these experiences drain mental energy. When mental energy is drained faster than it's replaced, we will experience significant daily ups and downs.

Capacity blockages are difficult to spot because we are so focused on the day to day – that's why an outside eye can see things that you cannot.

The Trap of Resource Maximization

I fell into the Trap of Resource Maximization. My "Yeah, but I've got three empty chairs there" comment is a perfect example of being caught in the trap.

Here's the trap … we want to maximize the utilization of everything we have.

That's fine if demand was even, but demand goes up and down.

If you have late afternoon and early evening appointments, my guess is they're booked way out. That's a time that people want to come in because people want to come in when they don't have to miss work.

It doesn't matter how many chairs you have empty at 2:00 or 11:00; it matters how many empty you have at 6:00. Most practices who are open at 6 don't have any empty chairs at 6:00.

We keep thinking, "Oh, we'll just get those people who want to come in at 6:00 to come in at 11:00 and everything will be great."

Think about that, you go to a McDonald's at 9:30 and there's a few people in there, but it's mostly empty. You go in at 12:30, the place is packed.

They try to have enough seats to have everybody be able to sit down and have a meal at 12:30, so they're way overbuilt for 9:30.

People want to come when they want to come, and you've got to be ready to serve people when they want to come.

We play great delusional mental games to deny being caught in the Trap of Resource Maximization.

We know that adding capacity will involve some level of increased chaos. If we add an additional team member, there's going to be some increased chaos. If we add a new technology, there's going to be some increased chaos. If we equip an additional room, there's going to be some increased chaos. We know that anytime you make change in the system, there's going to be some chaos

Second, adding capacity involves some risk. You hire an additional person who turns out to be a complete witch. They cause one of your good employees to leave. Every change includes some element of risk.

Thirdly, adding capacity risks my income ... Often when there is an investment made, it takes time to ramp up; sometimes it can negatively impact your income on a short-term basis.

Here are some questions to think about, to help determine if you have capacity issues in your practice:

1. Can you answer the phones? Every time the phone rings? Hardly anybody leaves a message anymore. If they call and they don't get an answer, very few will call back (especially when it comes to new patients.)

2. Can you make financial arrangements with every patient? Are you able to do the things it takes particularly with big case dentistry? Do you have the number of people and the time and the place to make good financial arrangements with every patient?

3. Can you maintain a low accounts receivable? Meaning, you're collecting the money.

4. Can you get new patients in fast? As you know, best definition of "fast" is how soon can you get here. But once you are looking at scheduling out more than two or three days, you're starting to sink. You really are.

    I have a group of practices that I'm working with in a southern city now, and they have wait times to get into their practice of three and four months. They think they're so great and doing so wonderful. Yet, they have all these patients that are leaving because they can't get in the appointment time in a timely manner, so they just leave. They are losing an amazing opportunity.

5. Can you do same-day dentistry? Does 30% to 50% of your daily revenue come from same-day dentistry? If it doesn't, you're probably out of capacity.

6. Is the doctor pressing for greater productivity and systemization? If the doctor is not pressing, it means she's fatigued and you're out of capacity.

7. Is the team pressing forward? If they're not, you're probably out of capacity (or you have the wrong team.)

Appointment availability for me is just the fastest, simplest way. If I'm a new patient and I call and ask, "When can I get in?" If the answer isn't "Today, tomorrow, at the very latest, the next day," you've got a problem. A practice with adequate capacity can tell a new patient emergency caller: "How soon can you get here?"

Here's some other statistics that you can use to see how you're doing capacity wise:

- Productivity per op, per month. This is a net production number. If you live in a place that has relatively standard fees -- about $20,000 per op, per month is average.

Dr. David Ahearn and I did a study. We were trying to determine if we could time when an additional op was going to be needed in a practice. We found it very complex to predict. We found that there are very, very, very few practices that get over $40,000 of net production per op, per month. Most were somewhere in the 30s, when they were running out of capacity and it's time to start getting additional ops. Net Productivity per full time employee equivalent per month. This one, it's easy to remember, it's the same. It's about $20,000. If you get up to $30,000 per

FTE, you probably are bumping into capacity issues.. You want to be efficient in utilizing the efforts of each team member. You don't want to run them ragged which leads to turnover.

My partner at the Team Training Institute, Wendy Briggs, teaches three roles of hygiene which includes the preventative therapist. And one of the ways that her hygienists can double their production is by doing same-day preventative services – like sealants.

We all know that if you re-appoint for a sealant, it turns into a missed or cancelled appointment. One of the requirements to be able to do same-day services is that you need every op prepped. In this case, it means we will need a curing light in each op. If you don't have that in each op, it means that people have to get up, bring it back (possibly wait because someone else is using it), and then put it away. This really kills time in a high-productive hygiene schedule – where there are no extra minutes to find.

We had a practice, who was working with one of our hygiene coaches, who wasn't progressing at the rate in which was expected. When we dug into why their hygiene productivity numbers were not growing, we quickly found out that the doctor was trying to save money by having his four hygienists share one curing light.

Now, how much does a curing light cost? About $1500? They have four hygienists so that would be an additional $4500 to provide each op with a curing light. Would you say that is expensive?

I say NO! Let's do the math. If you were able to add just four extra sealants in the hygienist's schedule per day … We would very quickly pay for those extra curing lights in a month, maybe two. Every month after that, it just gets better and better. Trying to save $4500, this doctor was walking away from tens of thousands of dollars.

Having capacity is important. Having what you need, where you need, and when you need makes a productive practice. If you don't, it's costing you a fortune and you don't realize it.

Overcoming Challenges

Sometimes overcoming capacity issues can be challenging. For example, they may require a tremendous investment to fix them.

I came to the realization when I needed one more person at the front desk that there was no room for one more person at the front desk.

I'm thinking, "Holy crap. I've got to do something very, very expensive to make room for one person in the right place."

Lucky for me, there was a small house next to my office for sale. I bought the house, made some minor modifications, and renamed it the Executive Suites.

We ran a computer line and a phone line over there, and we moved some people from our front desk to the Executive Suites.

All the incoming calls were answered there. The outgoing marketing calls, insurance verification, insurance filing, marketing, and our bookkeeping were all done from there. It took all pressure off the front desk.

The home cost about $40,000 so was far less expensive and far less chaotic than trying to remodel the office while working. We were lucky to have such a reasonable alternative, but we had to think outside of our four walls.

Why Are You Working Harder and Making Less Money?

Why You Should Always Be (Smartly) Marketing

Habit #7: Always be marketing

The highly successful practices all had a different mind-set about marketing and about new patients. Early in my career I had spent all this time building up great clinical skills which gave me the understanding, the knowledge, and the capability of doing large treatment plans and complex cases.

I felt like I was all dressed up with nowhere to go. I had all these capabilities, but I wasn't seeing the case acceptance that I wanted. I was going out to the market, trying to get more patients, trying to get the type of patients that I wanted.

No matter what kind of effort I did, I never seemed to get enough of the right type of patients. When I studied my successful mentors' practices I learned that they had a different way of looking at it.

Highly productive practices believe:

- Every patient is a good patient.
- The more the merrier.
- Market, track, measure, adjust and repeat.

Good patients

Nothing will get me fired up more than when someone says, "Well, I did x, y, and z and I got some patients, but they weren't good patients."

Every patient is a good patient.

Every patient has the opportunity to refer you more.

My initial deluded definition of a "good patient" -- and it was very, very unwise, to say the least -- was a patient who accepted all the care I thought they should have, paid for it, was nice, didn't ask questions, didn't challenge me, and then sent all their friends. That was what I thought a good patient was. I was wrong.

What I learned was that I was being judgmental. The highly productive dentists loved all the patients. They aren't looking for specific patients. They just want more patients. They took care of the each patient to the best of their ability.

I was being judgmental. I wasn't happy when people didn't accept my complex treatment plans or didn't want to do the entire treatment all at once. Well, patients could sense that I was being judgmental, whether I was trying to hide it or not. They sensed it and it had an impact on my practice.

When I stopped being judgmental and became grateful for every patient that came through the door, it changed my practice. All of a sudden, it was in a world of abundance, not a world of scarcity.

More the Merrier

Having a lot of patients is good. I love the quote from P. T. Barnum: "Nothing draws a crowd like a crowd."

When I visit an office for a consulting visit, I can tell how well the practice is doing with my eyes closed ... just by listening.

What do I listen for?

I listen for how friendly I'm greeted, first of all.

I listen to how much the phone is ringing.

I listen to the noise of dentistry going on in the back.

I listen to the conversations. Is it happy? Are people talking? Are people friendly?

Is it a place that I would want to be? Certainly, every patient is consciously or subconsciously doing the same evaluation.

Market, track, measure, adjust, and repeat

There are four components to a great marketing system:

1. Activity that leads to results
2. Carefully tracking results
3. Course correction
4. Spend more resources on what's working

Consider the 3 M's

To successfully market any business efficiently, you should consider the 3 M's of marketing. The market, the message, and the media.

Who is your market? When you are clear on this, it will give you 80% of your results.

I know of a practice that is a cosmetic reconstructive practice who advertises in airline magazines. They are bringing in patients from all over the United States as well as internationally. They have a specific market, and they have a specific market they are trying to attract. They need a world-class patient experience for this strategy to be sustainable. This example of niche marketing is a very high-risk strategy. Niche marketing often has a high cost of acquisition and produces fewer patients.

For most dentists the market is pretty simple to define. It is a mile radius around your practice. 80% of your patients will come from within a 5-mile radius. It is really easy to market and build a brand in a compact geographic area.

Once you know who you are trying to reach, the next question is, how do you reach them? There have never been more choices of media. The channels available to connect to your market keeps expanding and expanding and expanding. Channels might be television ads, radio ads, or newspaper ads. This might be direct mail, a website, or online ads. It might be Google Pay Per Click, it might be Facebook ads, or it might be connecting to people using other social media. The media you choose has to fit well with your market. It doesn't make sense to have paid media going out to the entire world when your market is a 5-mile radius. Determine what media you can use to get in front of the prospects that are in your market.

The last piece is the message -- what kind of things can you put in your marketing that will get them to take action? For some people, it's offering a very specific set of services. I have seen successful general ads. The type that says I am a dentist, I do these procedures, I am located here, and call this number now. I've seen advertising that has been successful in niches. For Invisalign. While more challenging, I've seen implant ads that have been successful. I have seen sedation ads that have been successful. I have seen discount ads that have been successful.

The messages will influence who you attract. There are few key pieces that you want to have in your message. You will at minimum want your message to answer these questions: Why should they come to see you? Why should they do it now? And how do they go about doing that?

One question that I often get revolves around "discounts" in marketing. One of these Apogee dentists I studied used a free exam and X-ray offer. He generated a large number of new patients which resulted in a large number of treatment plans, some of which were big cases. Many of those cases were really small. He was just trying to get volume. This allowed him to be treating the more complex cases while his associate dentists treated the simpler cases that were within their skill set. This strategy allowed him to become the most productive dentist that I am aware of.

I love this quote, "Half the money I spend on advertising is wasted, the trouble is I don't know which half." This was from John Wanamaker who was in Napoleon Hill's original mastermind group. I think it's really a clever quote.

Here is how you find out which half is working, and my hope is that you're going to have much more than half that's working – TRACKING. The purpose of tracking is to determine the best place to spend your marketing dollars.

The simplest way to determine what marketing activity influenced the patient to come in is to ask. You can do this on the phone or in person. There is no 100% accurate way of tracking. This method is easy, fast, cheap, and accurate enough.

I know people who have gone to great lengths to have a different phone number attached on every marketing effort. This method, it doesn't necessarily tell you how they heard about you; it only tells you where they found the number at the time they decided to call you.

Next, track the cost for each marketing activity. Let's say you have a couple of billboards up in town. Three new patients say that they learned of your office by your billboard. Once you know the number of new patients an activity is generating and the cost of that activity, you can compute a critical ratio. The ratio, cost of acquisition (COA), is the amount of dollars you spent on that marketing activity divided by the number of new patients you earned from that activity. This simple ratio tells you how much it costs to attract a new patient by the given activity.

Costs of acquisition can be all over the map. I was working with a practice whose target market was high-end big cases, and their cost of acquisition for one particular marketing activity was $4,000 per patient. One can easily see the problem if the cost of acquisition is high. The patients attracted will have to need, want, and be able to afford a lot of treatment. Otherwise, profitability will go down counter to the purpose of doing the marketing in the first place. Cost of acquisition, for most general bread-and-butter practices, have been rising for the last four or five years, and it's not unusual to see a cost of acquisition of $150/patient or more.

The next thing you want to track is the average new patient spend from every source. When they come to your office, how much are they spending? This will allow you to determine another important ratio, Return on Investment

(ROI.) Put simply, if we spend X on marketing, what are we getting in return? Let's say we spend $1,000 on postcards and we have 10 patients who come in and they spend a total of $100,000. We divide the total they spend ($100,000) by the number of responses (10), which give us $10,000 spent/new patient. We then divide the average amount they spent ($10,000) by the amount we spend on the marketing campaign ($1,000). $10,000/$1,000 = 10. The ROI is 10:1, meaning that for every dollar we spend in postcards, we received $10 back.

These figures help you make decisions on what you're going to do with your marketing spend. You want to maximize the ROI and reduce the COA.

One of the things I often hear is "My marketing's not working" or, more specifically, people will say marketing (in general) doesn't work. To that, I have a very simple answer. Think again. Marketing works. Good news-Bad news. Good news is it can draw in patients and help practices grow. Bad news is it can also help practices shrink.

Let me explain. If you have an amazing patient experience and you're generating a lot of direct referrals and you spend money on marketing, you're going to be bringing people into your practice who will have a great experience. These people will go out and tell their friends and family and refer more people. <u>This will speed up the rate of growth for your practice.</u>

Let's look at what happens if we don't have a great patient experience. You spend money on marketing, you draw in more people but those people are unhappy and they also go out and tell their friends and their family, and now they also talk about their experience on social media. <u>This will speed up the decline of your practice.</u>

I work with a practice that has very low patient satisfaction. The practice continues to spend more and more on marketing – thinking that this will solve their problem. All it is doing is bringing in more and more people, who go through a poor patient experience and leave unhappy. Their cost of acquisition keeps climbing, and their new patient numbers keep dropping as they continue to spend money to drive their practice into the ground.

Despite my explaining it to them and pointing out how they can reverse it, they still continue to do the same thing expecting different results – if they don't make changes soon, they will go bankrupt because they just don't understand what's happening.

Once you understand the cost of acquisition and return on investment, you can look at all the different ways that you're marketing your practice and all the different ways you're spending money to attract new patients and balance your spend. Start by listing everything you are doing, the cost of acquisition for that activity and the return on investment. Now rank them from best to worst. Drop the worst and spend more on what is working best.

One thing to remember, there's going to be a temptation to put all your eggs in one basket. One activity is going to pull greater than everything else. There was a time when direct mail was pulling very well in most markets. At that time, many people dropped everything else, put all their eggs into one basket. Then, when their competitors started to spend on direct mail and the effectiveness of it went down, they began to struggle because they didn't have another source for new patients.

Always be testing something new, always be dropping something off, but always be testing. I have seen people test the craziest stuff, and I'm always amazed at what will attract patients. For example, one practice paid for every fourth ad on the back of a Kroger grocery shopping receipt, and they are getting a 6:1 ROI. I've had other people who tried that and didn't get <u>any</u> response. So always be testing, always be tracking, always be dropping the ones that aren't pulling well, using some of the resources to test new things and some to do more of what is working.

But let's not forget **internal marketing**. Highly productive practices very carefully work on the five R's.

1. Referrals: What are we doing on a consistent basis to bring in referrals?

2. Recall: What are we doing to ensure that every patient is re-appointing for their next appointment?

3. Recovery: What are we doing to ensure that the schedules for and tomorrow are full?

4. Reactivation: How do we bring people back who have been away from the practice for a while?

5. Retention: What are we doing to ensure that patients have a good experience and stay with our practice?

One of the fastest ways to add a surge to your practice is through a reactivation campaign, and it's the second-best dollar you can spend (the first best dollar spend is on signage.) If you do not have a rolling reactivation campaign -- that's going out month after month reactivating patients who have dropped off for one reason or another -- you're really missing something powerful.

Internal marketing is really keeping you and your practice top of mind with patients. One practice that does this really well touches every patient once a month. They created different ways of touching people; through direct mail, through mass texts or mass e-mails. That kept them at the top of the mind for their patients.

I've got a wonderful car and a wonderful car dealer, and when it's time for anything to be done in my car, I get an e-mail, I'll get a call from the service department, I'll get a text from them. They're really good at making sure that my cars maintained perfectly. What's even more amazing is the maintenance of my car is under warranty, and so I don't have to pay for it, and they still work hard to make sure I get in there. That's taking care of their customers.

Another thing that I have seen work very well are condition-specific offers to current patients. You go through your database and identify patients who had been diagnosed with crowns that have not done them. Then you send out a "buy one, get one free" or "buy one, get the second one half off" direct mail piece to those people. One practice in a very affluent city had amazing results with this campaign. I was skeptical but the campaign drew patients in, and the practice achieved their most profitable month ever.

Why do they work? Most patients wanted to have their treatment but something got in the way. Life happened, and they didn't get it done. Having the reminder and a special offer now brought them in. This is also the basis of Invisalign days. You can go back and look for anybody who you've discussed Invisalign with, invite them to a special day, and have special pricing for that day. Those are often very, very successful. Your Invisalign rep will help you to make it successful.

Here's a truth. I do not know one way to get 100 new patients per month, but I do know 100 ways to get one. There is no magic bullet, there is nothing that works everywhere, there is nothing that works every time, and there's nothing that works forever. You need a system where you're trying, you're testing, you're measuring, you're bringing in the ones that win, and you're dropping off the ones that aren't winning. It's just that simple. Without this system your COA and ROI will be higher than necessary, your risk of spending unnecessarily will be high, and you will never be successful marketing.

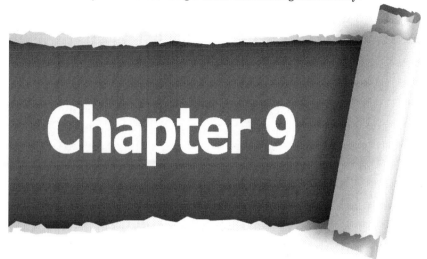

Know the Technology Rules

Habit #8: Know the technology rules

Highly productive practices use technology, but they use it differently than most. They use what I call an investment filter when deciding whether or not to invest in the new technology.

Investment Filter

The investment filter is the three key questions to ask when you're going to invest in technology:

1. "Does it add new capabilities? With this technology, can I do something that I can't do currently?"

2. "Will it increase treatment speed?"

129

Because speed matters to patients. For patients, the faster they can get done what needs to be done, as long as it's comfortable, the better.

3. "Does it improve the patient experience?"

I have some wonderful experiences with this. There was a day when micro abrasion, used as a treatment for small carious lesions, was the hot new thing. This technology is still used today and is very effective for certain types of lesions. But when these first came out, people were using them for all kinds of lesions. The selling point was you don't have to use anesthesia. Well, if it's a very, very, very, very small lesion, you don't, but if it has any size at all, you are going to be using anesthesia because the patient is going to be uncomfortable.

Did it increase treatment speed? No, it decreased it terribly. It's very, very slow. Did it improve the patient experience? No, you often had a very slow procedure that ended up getting more uncomfortable, as you get closer to having all the decay removed. You also made a mess with the abrasive particles all over everything. It was very, very messy. It decreased treatment speed and worsened the patient experience. In retrospect, it was not a good investment for me.

But here's the thing to think about. The people that are high, high producers, they buy stuff and they try it. If it works, great. If it doesn't work, they get rid of it and move on. I've seen so many practices that invested in a technology, and because they had sunk the cost, sunk the dollars into the cost of having that technology, they felt compelled to continue to use it even though it wasn't a positive for the practice or patient. This causing an increasing level of frustration which is using an increasing amount of mental energy (more on this later).

Dental equipment is cheap. It's just plain dirt cheap. I know when you get the bill and when you look at the cost, you get that quote, you think, "Man, that's a lot of money." It is a lot of money if you don't consider what you can produce with it. If you can add a new treatment, if you can increase treatment speed, if you can improve the patient experience and get more internal referrals, the cost of that equipment is very, very, very inexpensive.

A common thing in dental practices is to have a room that's not used very often. It might be called the overflow room, and it's used just every once in a while. Over time, all the stuff that doesn't work, all the stuff that nobody likes to use ends up in that room. Anything that's halfway decent gets plucked out of the room and scavenged. You end up with this room that nobody wants to use because nothing in it is easy to use, nothing works, and it is just a difficult room.

If you look at what it would cost to redo the entire room - maybe $20,000 or $25,000? Ask yourself, "What can you produce in a room every month?" $20,000 is not unusual. You could pay for the room in the very first month if you just got it functional.

The Third-Generation Rule

The first generation of any new technology is generally a beta version, so it doesn't necessarily work very well. It doesn't have all the features, it isn't user friendly and is generally highly expensive. The next generation gets better. The third generation is where it really starts to make sense.

If you look at any of the technologies that have come along, you'll see this effect ... where the first ones are big, they're clunky, they're expensive, they don't work very well, they're not very user friendly, and then it gets better from there. I've always used the third-generation rule. When I see something in a magazine or at a conference that looks brand new and looks really great, I gather information on it and put it into a folder named "Maybe later" and then just track what happens as it comes to the next generation.

Next, I start looking for practices that are using the new gizmo. If I don't find somebody who's using it and using it effectively, I don't want it. The gizmo is simply not ready yet. So I'll wait for the next generation and do the same thing, see if I can find a practice that's using it effectively.

When it comes to implementation on technology, highly productive doctors focused on the <u>best use</u> of that technology, not every use of the technology.

When I look at things, like a practice management software, there are a thousand things that a practice management software can do. There is very rarely a practice that's using all of the capabilities of any practice management software system, and that's just fine. Focus on the best use, not every use.

I know people who have gotten CAD/CAM technology and have started out doing posterior restorations, and as they took more training, they started doing anterior restorations, and some even doing veneers. I've seen practices get so focused on using the technology to its fullest that they often lose sight of the best use.

In my opinion -- and I know I'll offend some people when I say this -- CAD/CAM technology for porcelain veneers is not a great technology. In my humble opinion, appearance is not what can be done with stackable porcelain. Can you do it? Yes, you can do it. Is it the best use for that technology? In my opinion, it's not. So don't try to use technology for everything; find its best use and stick with that.

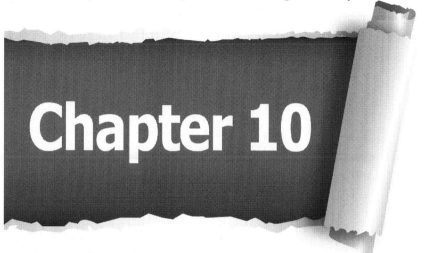

What Patients Really Want vs. Need vs. You Want

Habit #9: Wants, needs, want

Highly productive dentists take the time to clearly understand what their patients want.

Steve Jobs said:

"It's not the job of the customer to know what they want."

And that may be true in technology, but I like to say in dentistry, it is the dentist's job to **know** what they want -- very important.

I've seen so many times when there was a disconnect or a mismatch between where the patient was headed and where the dentist was headed, and it's bound to end up in a fail.

A very common thing that I observe looks like this… the dentist walks into the room, there's some minor small talk, the dentist does an exam, the dentist tells the patient what they need, dentist leaves the room, and now the financial coordinator's job is to try to get this patient to accept care that the patient really didn't want.

The dentist never really waited, listened, or found out what the patient wanted.

I see it all the time.

I learned this from a dentist in Canada. He had a very unique way of talking to patients about treatment.

First of all, he never did an exam until the treatment plan was done. When I tell people that, they are like, "What are you talking about? That doesn't make sense; that's nuts." It's not nuts.

The treatment plan was derived from conversation with the patient. While the patient is looking at photos of their own mouth a conversation is happening about what the patient wants. Before the exam was ever done, this dentist knew exactly where the treatment plan was going. Now, he may have observed a minor restoration here or there during the exam that added to the treatment plan, but the general direction of treatment was decided upon, and mentally bought, before the exam was ever done.

This amazing dentist never "told" his patients what they needed. There was no "telling" in his patient experience. What he did was he asked excellent questions to **guide the patient to make decisions.** It's a very, very unique system of guiding patients using powerful questions. With questions, he helped patients get a clue both of what's available and what they need. I go through this process and the 'power questions' to ask in The Art of Selling-High End Dentistry Training available at www.TheTeamTrainingInstitute.com

"If you want your kids to do what you tell them, find out what they are going to do and tell them to do it."

I think that's a quote from Abraham Lincoln, and it's so true. It's the same thing with patients. Find out what the patients want before you ever put any ideas in their head. With good questions and a good system of helping people see, feel, and sense what was going on in their mouth you never need to tell them anything. You guide them with questions to help them understand what they need. You use questions to help them guide you to what they want.

You Get One Shot at It

I was visiting a practice in Texas with one of the most productive dentists that I know. With the amount that he was producing each month, I thought he was seeing a lot of high-end patients – boy, was I wrong. There was a patient who came in who only had three teeth left, they're all loose, and the patient wanted the middle of the three teeth left taken out. This dentist took that tooth out and said, "Come on back when you're ready to do something with those other two." He did it quickly and efficiently and without judgment. It was such an eye-opener for me. I began to understand that if you meet patients where they are and with what they want, you are going to be far more successful.

You only get one shot at helping them understand what is possible, and if you don't bring them to your way of thinking, then it's your job to happily, humbly, cheerfully, and with gratitude give them what they want.

This was very hard for me to accept. If they didn't want what I wanted for them, I tried to change their mind. I judged them. I thought they weren't a "good patient."

I now look back on it. I was controlling. I was arrogant. I was demeaning to them. I offended them.

It wasn't my intention. I wanted to help them sincerely.

But how I was coming across was arrogant and demeaning, and people left without making an appointment.

It's amazing. When I got this right, people did make appointments. They could afford the treatment. They didn't need to ask their spouse before moving forward.

This one awareness changed my practice profoundly.

Why Are You Working Harder and Making Less Money?

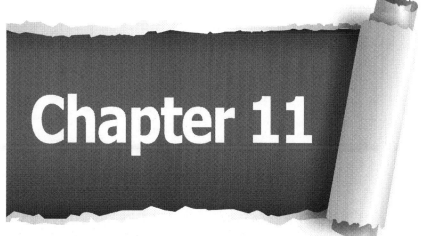

Why the Successful Are Always Willing to Try Everything

Habit #10: Understand Research and Development

Highly productive dentists do a lot of research and development. They try EVERYTHING. They also know when to let go and when it's not working.

I love this quote, "*Ancora imparo,*" which is Latin for "I am still learning." Michelangelo scribed that into one of his books when he was 80 years old. One of the most brilliant men in the history of the world was still learning when he was at that age.

Highly Successful Learners

Great learners, first, study their craft. These are just few clinical course series that I went through: the Dawson Center, Frank Spear, The Misch Implant Institute, Ross Nash's esthetic continuum, and the AGD Mastership series.

The highly successful doctors I studied all continued to improve their treatment abilities. They developed the capacity to understand complex cases. They developed the capacity to do more comprehensive care. They weren't trying to do it on everybody; instead, it was just one tool in their tool belt, ready and available for those who wanted it.

Highly Successful Readers

Great learners not only study their craft, they learn from others. They're voracious readers, they watch videos, listen to CDs in their car, listen to podcasts, read books, and they're learning things like business, leadership, management, marketing, and personal development.

I know of at least ten people in my circle of friends who read at least one book every week. I continue to learn so many fantastic things, so many concepts I would have never understood if I didn't have that one habit.

Learning from Aliens

The other thing that these highly successful dentists did is that they learned from "aliens." I don't mean the men from outer space; I mean industries that are not dental.

Here are some ways that these practices learned from aliens. The Disney Institute and Ritz-Carlton have great programs on the customer experience and customer satisfaction. I've been through both, and I highly recommend them. They're well done, well thought out, and really will give you a great foundation. My recommendation is if you go to either one of these, take as many of your team as you possibly can. Patient satisfaction is a team effort and far easier when the entire team has the training.

Going through building a customer-oriented culture is an experience; it's what these organizations do best. Zappos, known for their great company culture, has a program that you can go to about building a company culture.

One of the practices that was in this group did something that I thought was extremely innovative. They learned that there was a pharmacy that had an after-hours pickup for pharmacy refills. You could call in a prescription, and they would give you a code to pick it up. They would fill the refill, and they would put it into a lockbox where you could pick it up 24 hours a day.

143

I am sure there are a lot of rules and regulations to contend with in order to make this innovative service happen. A dental practice took this idea and used it to provide their patients with their whitening trays. When patients came in for their cleanings, if they wanted Whitening for Life™, they could take their impressions, give them the materials and instructions and a code for their lockbox. Once the trays were completed, the patient would come back, click their number in, and pull out their trays.

It eliminated the second visit so that the practice wasn't burning chair time, and it allowed the patient to get them any time 24 hours a day. The patient didn't have to schedule a second appointment; they picked up their trays whenever it was convenient. A great example of learning from aliens.

Practice Visits

Highly successful dentists learn from each other. I have seen the insides of over 263 different practices. I can tell you that I learn something new from each one.

In one practice visit, I learned something that made my personal productivity go up $40,000 the very next month!

It was a little thing but it was an important thing for me, and I would have never figured it out on my own.

Copy Others

"If someone's doing it successfully, it's probably possible."

Now, there were things that were very successful in other practices that I tried to implement in mine and, for whatever reason, didn't work as well in mine as it had in the original.

That happens. But, nonetheless, there are things I tried in my practice that I wouldn't have thought would have worked which worked really well.

Why Are You Working Harder and Making Less Money?

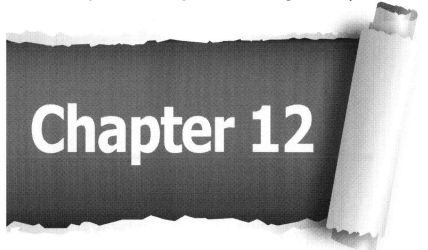

Winning the Mental Game

Habit #11: Winning the Mental Game

Highly successful dentists understand that life is a mental game. It's quite simply making sure that you are prepared mentally every day and that you are keeping your mental energy in check.

In dentistry, what do we run out of first, mental energy or physical energy? Mental energy. I quickly learned how to conserve mental energy which is one of the key pieces to becoming highly productive.

In my training program Clinical Explosion and in our Double Your Production Membership, I talk a lot about the concept of mental energy and all the little ways that you can conserve and replenish that energy in order to become highly productive. **<u>High productivity is only 1/6th about</u>**

your actual clinical skills and 5/6th about everything else.

One of the ways of saving mental energy is through delegation. Now, I mean clinical delegation, where the dentist is only doing those things that dentists are trained to do and delegating everything else. You should train your teams to do the things allowed by your state's laws. The laws in states vary, and in the state where I used to live, Kentucky, dental assistants who have earned the expanded function status can place restorative material. Hygienists can provide anesthesia. Think of it. Hygienist numbs, dentist preps, assistants finish the restoration. Amazingly efficient.

That's great delegation. Now, the dentist isn't burning mental energy placing the restorative material, adjusting it, making sure the contact's perfect, making sure there's no overhangs, etc.

All those things that go into the placement of restorative material, a dentist doesn't have to burn mental energy to do that. Now, that may be an extreme example, but other places that I see that dentists delegate, where allowed is placement of retraction cord, making temporary restorations, and impressions. Where hygienists are allowed to do anesthesia, that certainly can and should be delegated.

Everything that a dentist doesn't have to do should be delegated. Now, does that mean a dentist never is giving an injection? No, it doesn't work out that way in the real flow of a clinical practice. But to the degree that you can, you're delegating all clinical things allowed. You're also delegating all the non-clinical things as well.

I see dentists still today who are involved in the ordering of supplies. That makes absolutely no sense. You can have someone who is making $15 an hour doing that.

Highly productive dentists are usually excellent teachers. They help their teams understand the context to use in making decisions. The better your team can make decisions, the less you'll have to. Decision making is a huge mental energy-burner.

Another huge burner of mental energy is *schedule-watchers.* I know this sounds funny -- and you know who you are if you are one -- that you're watching the schedule trying to figure out, "Will this work? Will this not work?" Really trying to talk yourself out of the treatment that's on the schedule.

What usually happens is you see a place in the schedule where it's going to be tight, you're not sure it's going to work, and now you worry about it, and you're just draining mental energy. I can go into any practice in the United States, and I can find out who the schedule-maniacs are --

the ones who watch the schedule all the time and stress about whether it's going to work or not.

If it's a multi-doctor practice, they are generally the least productive doctors in the practice. Schedule-maniacs, clock-watchers, it doesn't work. Schedule watching is a huge drain on mental energy. Get over it, help your team understand the context on how to make schedule decisions, and stay out of it -- they'll work it out.

When I understood that, and I stopped watching our schedule, I was up $40,000 a month.

It's so simple but it's so profound.

I was a schedule-watcher.

What I learned was that there was an inverse proportion of schedule watching to productivity.

My practice had someone watching the schedule saying, "Oh, this won't work here, this won't work here, and this won't work here." That person was no longer me. I learned it's not my job.

My job is to go where they tell me to go. My job is not to watch the schedule.

I learned this at a visit to the office of Dr. Vince Monticciolo. He has a whiteboard located outside the op near the center of his practice. On the whiteboard are columns for room, procedure and anesthesia. The team updates the whiteboard with information on where the doctor is to go next.

He finishes treating a patient, walks out, and immediately looks at the whiteboard. He sees Room Number 3, we're doing seven crowns, and the patient is anesthetized. Room Number 5 needs a hygiene exam.

Now, he has not looked at the schedule. He doesn't know what his schedule is. He doesn't need to know what his schedule is.

All he needs to know is where to go next because if he knows everything on the schedule and what's going on and what's going in this room, in this room, in this room, he's burning mental energy.

He walks out and can see Room 3 is seven crowns with anesthesia and Room 5 needs a hygiene exam which will likely take two minutes.

He might do this two-minute thing, then go do the crowns.

It doesn't eliminate the thought process, but all he does is look at what's on the board and goes and does the next thing.

He never looks at the schedule.

This one thing improved my productivity $40,000 the very next month.

I was so busy thinking about what's going on here and what's going on there and trying to orchestrate it all. I didn't need to do that; the team can do that.

I was burning all this very, very valuable mental energy.

If you can spend 90% of your time doing only the things that dentists have to do, another 10% of time doing training, giving context, and making decisions -- only high-level decisions -- that's when you get to be the most productive.

One of the dentists in this group that I was studying, had a rule: His office manager could make decisions that were going to cost less than $50,000. If it was over $50,000, she had to talk to him.

Now, did that happen without him training? No. Did it happen without him helping that person have a lot of context on how to make decisions? No, it didn't. It took time to get there. But if you don't start, you will never get there.

You want to hang on to every last bit of mental energy you possibly can.

Work Hard, Play Hard

The next part of the mental game is work hard, play hard.

Highly successful dentists (and people for that matter), when they're at work, they work really hard. When they stop working, they're done working.

They don't work all the time. They don't bring stuff home and work on it. If they do, there's a start point and there's a stop point.

If you are not careful, over time this work kind of just goes on and on. There's never a start point and a stop point.

Rest, relaxation, and play all build mental energy.

If you don't have the play time, you don't have the mental energy to maximize your work time.

Mental energy is the most valuable resource that you have. Work hard but shut it off and have fun.

What Do You Do Now?

Once I learned these 11 habits, I set out to IMPLENT each into my practice. Without implementation, there will never be high productivity.

I took these habits and created five steps that any doctor can use to double their production and grow their practice. I outline the entire system in the book *The Ultimate Guide to Doubling and Tripling Your Dental Practice Production* (available on Amazon or at www.TheTeamTrainingInstitute.com)

This is what the Team Training Institute specializes in -- helping dental practices maximize their production, maximize their team's efforts, and provide their patients with a world-class experience that they can't help but tell their friends and family about.

Much of this starts with Chapter 1 and creating a clear vision as this will drive everything and every decision in your practice.

And it starts with celebrating … you've made it to the end of the book, a sign that you have what it takes to become a highly productive, highly successful dentist.

Not everyone will make it this far. I have read that only 20% of people finish what they start – which I am sure is an overestimation at 20%.

As I said in the beginning, becoming highly successful is all about a mind-set. A commitment to do what it takes to becoming successful. But you don't have to do it alone.

The most successful people don't try to do this alone. They rely on mentors, coaches, and those who have done it before them – that is the quickest path to success.

There are two ways that I can help you, if you are looking for the next steps:

1. You can participate in a Vision Day where you come out and spend a day with me where I will help you create clarity and find your vision – which will give you the starting point for all decisions in your practice. To find out more about this day, email me at johnmeis@theteamtraininginstitute.com with "vision day" in the subject line.

2. Before doing any more marketing, you need to determine if it's driving your practice to growth or decline. Our production specialists can analyze your practice and provide you with the right road map for your practice growth. You can set up a private road map customization by emailing me at johnmeis@theteamtraininginstitute.com or by going to www.DoubleYourProductionRoadmap.com

About the Author

Dr. Meis is a fourth-generation dentist.

His father and his father's father and his father's father's father were all dentists.

So he's been said to have "dentistry in his blood" … literally.

He is an international speaker, trainer, coach, and author. He is an innovator in practice management, marketing, leadership, and team development.

When he was practicing, he was in the top 1% of producers in the United States. He tripled his practice in just four years and multiplied his one practice into 12.

Dr. Meis has played a key role -- visiting, coaching and innovating on the ground -- inside over 180 dental practices.

He's also a Fellow in the Academy of General Dentistry (FAGD) and a Diplomate of the International Congress of Oral Implantologists (DICOI).

Free Resources Just For Book Readers!

Because this topic is so important to the Dental Community and because everyone learns differently, we have created a special area for readers of this book.

The great news is access to this area is completely free.

You can register and receive free access at...

www.11HabitsToolkit.com

Here's what you will find when you register for your free access...

✴ All of the downloadable resources mentioned throughout the book.

✴ 3 advanced video trainings on the 11 Secrets of Highly Successful Dentists

✴ BONUS Video Training: What Got You To Where You Are Today Won't Get You To Where You Want To Go Tomorrow

Simply register to receive free access at:

www.11HabitsToolkit.com

Made in the USA
Middletown, DE
08 September 2018